Volume 2

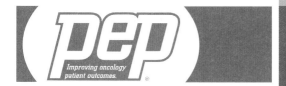

Oncology Nursing Society

PUTTING

EVIDENCE *INTO*

PRACTICE

Improving Oncology Patient Outcomes

EDITED BY

Linda H. Eaton, MN, RN, AOCN®, Janelle M. Tipton, MSN, RN, AOCN®, and Margaret Irwin, PhD, RN, MN

Oncology Nursing Society
Pittsburgh, Pennsylvania

ONS Publications Department

Interim Publisher and Director of Publications: Barbara Sigler, RN, MNEd
Managing Editor: Lisa M. George, BA
Technical Content Editor: Angela D. Klimaszewski, RN, MSN
Staff Editor II: Amy Nicoletti, BA
Copy Editor: Laura Pinchot, BA
Graphic Designer: Dany Sjoen

Putting Evidence Into Practice: Improving Oncology Patient Outcomes, Volume 2

Library of Congress Control Number: 2009926935
ISBN 978-1-935864-04-2

Publisher's Note

Printed in the United States of America

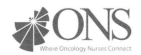

Oncology Nursing Society
Integrity • Innovation • Stewardship • Advocacy • Excellence • Inclusiveness

Contributors

Editors

Linda H. Eaton, MN, RN, AOCN®
Research Nurse
University of Washington School of Nursing
Seattle, Washington
Author (Chapter 1)

Janelle M. Tipton, MSN, RN, AOCN®
Oncology Clinical Nurse Specialist
University of Toledo Medical Center
Toledo, Ohio
Author (Chapter 1)

Margaret Irwin, PhD, RN, MN
Research Associate
Research Department
Oncology Nursing Society
Pittsburgh, Pennsylvania
Author (Chapter 1)

Chapter Editors

Deborah Hutchinson Allen, MSN, CNS, FNP-
    BC, AOCNP®
Clinical Nurse Specialist, Inpatient Oncology
Duke University Medical Center
Durham, North Carolina
*Chapter 2; Cognitive Impairment PEP
    Resource*

Tara Baney, RN, MS, ANP-BC, AOCN®
Oncology Nurse Practitioner
Penn State Hershey Medical Group
State College, Pennsylvania
Chapter 4; Radiodermatitis PEP Resource

Marcelle Kaplan, RN, MS, AOCN®, CBCN®
Breast Oncology Clinical Nurse Specialist
    and Consultant
Merrick, New York
Chapter 3; Hot Flashes PEP Resource

Jeanene (Gigi) Robison, MSN, RN, AOCN®
Oncology Clinical Nurse Specialist
The Christ Hospital
Cincinnati, Ohio
Chapter 5; Skin Reactions PEP Resource

Authors

Rachel Behrendt, DNP, MSN, APN-C, AOCNS®
Senior Director, Staff Development and Magnet Recognition Program®
Thomas Jefferson University Hospital
Philadelphia, Pennsylvania
Cognitive Impairment PEP Resource

Kathleen Bell, RN, MSN, OCN®
Clinical Nurse Specialist
Grand Rapids, Michigan
Radiodermatitis PEP Resource

Patricia Bieck, RN, BSN, OCN®
Senior Staff Nurse III, Safety Nurse Radiation Oncology
James P. Wilmot Cancer Center
University of Rochester
Rochester, New York
Radiodermatitis PEP Resource

Susan Bruce, RN, MSN, OCN®
Oncology Clinical Nurse Specialist
Duke Raleigh Cancer Center
Raleigh, North Carolina
Radiodermatitis PEP Resource

Julie Carlson, MSN, RN, APN, AOCNS®
Oncology Clinical Nurse Specialist
OSF Saint Anthony Medical Center
Rockford, Illinois
Skin Reactions PEP Resource

Therese Carpizo, MSN, RN, AOCN®
Adjunct Faculty, Clinical and Laboratory Instructor
Elgin Community College
Elgin, Illinois
Skin Reactions PEP Resource

Diane Cope, RN, PhD, ARNP-BC, AOCNP®
Oncology Nurse Practitioner
Florida Cancer Specialists
Fort Myers, Florida
Hot Flashes PEP Resource

Deborah Feight, RN, MSN, CNS, AOCN®
Radiation Oncology Clinical Nurse Specialist
Northwest Ohio Oncology Center/Toledo Radiation Oncology
Toledo, Ohio
Radiodermatitis PEP Resource

Ann Fuhrman, BSN, RN, OCN®
Staff Nurse, Inpatient Oncology Unit
The Christ Hospital
Cincinnati, Ohio
Skin Reactions PEP Resource

Phyllis Gagnon, RN, BSN, OCN®
Oncology Clinical Nurse and Long-Term Cancer Survivor
Radiation Oncology Center
Inova Loudoun Hospital
Leesburg, Virginia
Cognitive Impairment PEP Resource

Marilyn Haas, PhD, RN, CNS, ANP-C
Nurse Practitioner
CarePartners and Carolina Clinical Consultant
Asheville, North Carolina
Radiodermatitis PEP Resource

Stacey Hill, RN, BSN
Staff Nurse
Tennessee Valley Gynecologic Oncology
Huntsville, Alabama
Hot Flashes PEP Resource

Marcie Jacobson, RN, BSN, OCN®
Head Nurse
Florida Cancer Specialists
Fort Myers, Florida
Hot Flashes PEP Resource

Catherine Jansen, PhD, RN, CNS, OCN®
Oncology Clinical Nurse Specialist
Kaiser Permanente Medical Center
San Francisco, California
Cognitive Impairment PEP Resource

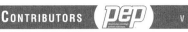

Elizabeth Keating, RN, MS, NP, CBCN®
Oncology Nurse Practitioner
University of Massachusetts Memorial Medical Center
Worcester, Massachusetts
Hot Flashes PEP Resource

Suzanne Mahon, RN, DNSc, AOCN®, APNG
Professor
Division of Hematology/Oncology, Department of Internal Medicine
Professor, Adult Nursing, School of Nursing
Saint Louis University
St. Louis, Missouri
Hot Flashes PEP Resource

Maurene McQuestion, RN, BScN, MSc, CON(C)
Clinical Nurse Specialist, Advanced Practice Nurse
Radiation Medicine Program
Princess Margaret Hospital University Health Network
Toronto, Ontario, Canada
Radiodermatitis PEP Resource

Denise Portz, BSN, RN, OCN®
Medical Oncology Nursing Team Leader
Regional Cancer Center-Waukesha Memorial Hospital
Waukesha, Wisconsin
Skin Reactions PEP Resource

Rosalina M. Schiavone, RN, BSN, OCN®
Clinician III Treatment Room Nurse
Alta Bates Summit Comprehensive Cancer Center
Berkeley, California
Cognitive Impairment PEP Resource

Gary Shelton, MSN, ANP-BC, RN, AOCNP®
Adult Health Nurse Practitioner and Oncology Clinical Nurse Specialist
New York University Langone Medical Center and Comprehensive Cancer Center
New York, New York
Skin Reactions PEP Resource

Diane Von Ah, PhD, RN
Assistant Professor
Robert Wood Johnson Nurse Faculty Scholar
Indiana University School of Nursing
Indianapolis, Indiana
Cognitive Impairment PEP Resource

Linda Weis-Smith, RN, OCN®
Staff Nurse
Ministry Saint Joseph's Hospital
Marshfield, Wisconsin
Radiodermatitis PEP Resource

Loretta A. Williams, PhD, RN, AOCN®
Assistant Professor, Department of Symptom Research
University of Texas MD Anderson Cancer Center
Houston, Texas
Skin Reactions PEP Resource

Jennifer Wulff, RN, MN, ARNP, AOCNP®
Advanced Practice Nurse
The Ben and Catherine Ivy Center for Advanced Brain Tumor Treatment
Swedish Neuroscience Institute
Seattle, Washington
Cognitive Impairment PEP Resource

Librarians:
Andy Hickner, MSI
Administrative Specialist
Patient Safety Enhancement Program
University of Michigan Medical School
Ann Arbor, Michigan
Hot Flashes PEP Resource

Mark Vrabel, MLS, AHIP, ELS
Information Resources Supervisor
Library and Archives Department
Oncology Nursing Society
Pittsburgh, Pennsylvania
Cognitive Impairment PEP Resource; Hot Flashes PEP Resource; Radiodermatitis PEP Resource; Skin Reactions PEP Resource

Oncology Nursing Society Staff Support

Margaret Irwin, PhD, RN, MN
Research Associate
Research Department
Oncology Nursing Society
Pittsburgh, Pennsylvania
*Cognitive Impairment PEP Resource, Radio-
dermatitis PEP Resource,
Skin Reactions PEP Resource*

Kristen Fessele, RN, MSN, ANP-BC, AOCN®
Research Associate
Research Department
Oncology Nursing Society
Pittsburgh, Pennsylvania
*Hot Flashes PEP Resource; Skin Reactions
PEP Resource*

Field Reviewers

Darcy Burbage, RN, MSN, AOCN®, CBCN®
Survivorship Nurse Navigator
Helen F. Graham Cancer Center
Newark, Delaware
Hot Flashes PEP Resource

Kathy D. Burns, RN, MSN, OCN®
Manager of Radiation Oncology Nursing
Hartford Hospital
Hartford, Connecticut
Radiodermatitis PEP Resource

Ellen DeLuca, PhD, RN
Associate Professor of Nursing
Lynchburg College
Lynchburg, Virginia
Hot Flashes PEP Resource

Sandra E. Kurtin, RN, MS, AOCN®, ANP-C
Hematology/Oncology Nurse Practitioner
Arizona Cancer Center
Clinical Assistant Professor of Nursing and
Assistant Professor of Medicine
University of Arizona
Tucson, Arizona
Skin Reactions PEP Resource

Jamie S. Myers, PhD, RN, AOCN®
Volunteer Faculty
University of Kansas School of Nursing
Kansas City, Kansas
Cognitive Impairment PEP Resource

Emily K. Olson, NP
Nurse Practitioner
The Tucker Gosnell Center for Gastrointesti-
nal Cancers
Massachusetts General Hospital
Boston, Massachusetts
Skin Reactions PEP Resource

Karen Scanlon Henry, MSN, ARNP, FNP-BC
Nurse Practitioner, Radiation Oncology
University of Miami
Miami, Florida
Radiodermatitis PEP Resource

Brenda Shelton, MS, RN, CCRN, AOCN®
Clinical Nurse Specialist
Sidney Kimmel Comprehensive Cancer
Center at Johns Hopkins
Baltimore, Maryland
Skin Reactions PEP Resource

Agnes Wong, RN, MS, OCN®
Staff Nurse
Kaiser Permanente Medical Center
San Francisco, California
Cognitive Impairment PEP Resource

Disclosure

Editors and authors of books and guidelines provided by the Oncology Nursing Society are expected to disclose to the readers any significant financial interest or other relationships with the manufacturer(s) of any commercial products.

A vested interest may be considered to exist if a contributor is affiliated with or has a financial interest in commercial organizations that may have a direct or indirect interest in the subject matter. A "financial interest" may include, but is not limited to, being a shareholder in the organization; being an employee of the commercial organization; serving on an organization's speakers bureau; or receiving research from the organization. An "affiliation" may be holding a position on an advisory board or some other role of benefit to the commercial organization. Vested interest statements appear in the front matter for each publication.

Contributors are expected to disclose any unlabeled or investigational use of products discussed in their content. This information is acknowledged solely for the information of the readers.

The contributors provided the following disclosure and vested interest information:

Rachel Behrendt, RN, DNP, APN-C, AOCNS®: Mader Communications, Carmel Pharma, and Care Fusion, consultant or advisory role; Carmel Pharma, honoraria

Kathleen E. Bell, RN, MSN, OCN®, Medimark and American Society of Therapeutic Radiation Oncology, honoraria

Contents

CHAPTER 1

PEP Up Your Practice:
Expanding the Putting Evidence Into Practice Resources

Linda H. Eaton, MN, RN, AOCN®,
Janelle M. Tipton, MSN, RN, AOCN®,
and Margaret Irwin, PhD, RN, MN

Introduction

The Oncology Nursing Society (ONS) Putting Evidence Into Practice (PEP) Resources are essential for facilitating the use of evidence-based oncology nursing interventions in practice. The ONS PEP Resources' purpose is to provide the best scientific evidence for improving cancer care and patient-centered outcomes.

Oncology Nursing Society PEP Resources

The development of the ONS PEP Resources was a result of the Society's nursing-sensitive patient outcomes and evidence-based practice (EBP) work (see Table 1-1). ONS PEP Resources for 16 topics are available in *Putting Evidence Into Practice: Improving Oncology Patient Outcomes* (Eaton & Tipton, 2009). The book stresses the importance of measuring the clinical problem to determine the effectiveness of the evidence-based interventions and provides examples of measurement tools.

Nursing interventions that have been empirically tested are identified in the ONS PEP Resources. Interventions supported by expert opinion are also included. If no evidence is available for an intervention, it will not be found in the ONS PEP Resource.

This second volume of *Putting Evidence Into Practice* is a supplement to the 2009 book and provides resources in four new topic areas:
• Cognitive impairment
• Hot flashes
• Radiodermatitis
• Skin reactions.

Table 1-1. History of Oncology Nursing Society (ONS) Activities and Resources Related to Nursing-Sensitive Patient Outcomes and Evidence-Based Practice	
Year	**ONS Activities and Resources**
1998	**Outcomes State-of-the-Knowledge Conference** • The conference defined oncology nursing-sensitive patient outcomes (NSPOs) and provided direction for the promotion of evidence-based practice in both clinical practice and research.
2002	**Evidence-Based Practice Resource Area** • The Web site (www.ons.org/Research) provides general information, strategies, and resources for using evidence to solve clinical problems.
2003	**Outcomes Project Team** • The team recommended development of an ONS white paper on NSPOs and development of resources for measuring specific NSPOs. The Outcomes Project Team also created the five-year ONS NSPO Strategic Plan.
2004	**Measurement Summaries** • Internet resources (www.ons.org/Research/PEP) were created for measuring specific NSPOs for each PEP topic. **Nursing-Sensitive Patient Outcomes Advanced Practice Nursing (APN) Retreat** • APN retreat attendees reviewed evidence-based measurement summaries. • Attendees recommended the development of evidence-based resources that identify nursing interventions based on the best available evidence with the goal of improving NSPOs.
2005	**Nursing-Sensitive Patient Outcomes White Paper** • Barbara Given, PhD, RN, FAAN, and Paula Sherwood, PhD, RN, CNRN, authored this defining document.
2006	**PEP Resources: Volume 1** • Chemotherapy-Induced Nausea and Vomiting, Fatigue, Prevention of Infection, and Sleep-Wake Disturbances were included. **Outcomes Resource Area** • The Web site (www.ons.org/Research) provides information on NSPOs, evidence-based measurement summaries, and ONS PEP Resources.
2007	**PEP Resources: Volumes 2 and 3** • Caregiver Burden, Constipation, Depression, Dyspnea, Mucositis, Pain, Peripheral Neuropathy, and Prevention of Bleeding resources were released.
2008	**PEP Resources: Volume 4** • Anorexia, Anxiety, Diarrhea, and Lymphedema resources were released.
2009	***Putting Evidence Into Practice: Improving Oncology Patient Outcomes*** • ONS published the text that included 16 ONS PEP topics and updated evidence-based nursing interventions. • Examples of clinical measurement tools for assessing each PEP topic, case studies, and information on implementing the ONS PEP Resources in practice were included in this book.

(Continued on next page)

Table 1-1. History of Oncology Nursing Society (ONS) Activities and Resources Related to Nursing-Sensitive Patient Outcomes and Evidence-Based Practice *(Continued)*	
Year	**ONS Activities and Resources**
2011	***Putting Evidence Into Practice: Improving Oncology Patient Outcomes***, Volume 2 • Four new ONS PEP topics: Cognitive Impairment, Hot Flashes, Radiodermatitis, and Skin Effects are included in this book. • Evidence-based nursing interventions, description of clinical measurement tools, and case studies are also features. • Identification of prevention, late effects, and survivorship issues are new to this book.

The following areas of the PEP development process and resources have been enhanced with this current volume.

• The content of chapters has been expanded to include prevention, late effects and survivorship issues, areas for research, and documentation of the literature search strategy used.
  – As part of the ONS identification of cancer survivorship as a priority area, the ONS Survivorship Think Tank (2009) identified incorporation of survivorship issues into PEP Resources as part of the ONS Cancer Survivorship Initiatives Roadmap. Each chapter incorporates current knowledge regarding survivorship issues and late effects related to the topic.
  – The Evidence-Based Practice Advisory Group to the ONS Research Team suggested that identification of areas for future nursing research for each PEP topic would be useful. Because PEP teams are immersed in the research and other literature for each topic, they are in a good position to identify knowledge gaps in the existing literature that suggest research opportunities and needs. Areas for research identified by each team are included.
  – The process used for the review of the literature in a format that can be reproduced is incorporated for each topic. This has been written in the patient/problem, intervention, comparison, and outcome (commonly known as PICO) format.
• PEP teams adopted the Institute of Medicine and National Guideline Clearinghouse definition and inclusion criteria of clinical practice guidelines for inclusion as guidelines in PEP Resources. Basic definitions and criteria are shown in Figure 1-1. Materials that were based primarily on consensus rather than strict evaluation of evidence have been incorporated into PEP materials as "expert opinion" rather than "guidelines" where appropriate. Full text of the definition and criteria used can be found at http://guidelines.gov/about/inclusion-criteria.aspx.
• PEP teams adopted the general standard to exclude the use of "gray" literature, such as abstracts or correspondence, in the summary of evidence. Such material is only included where it is the only information found related to interventions currently being used in clinical practice.

Figure 1-1. Guidelines Definition and Inclusion Criteria

Definition
Systematically developed statements to assist decisions about appropriate health care for specific clinical circumstances

Criteria for Inclusion as Clinical Guidelines
- Includes systematically developed recommendations, strategy, or information that assists healthcare practitioners and patients to make decisions about appropriate care.
- Produced under the auspices of medical specialty associations, relevant professional societies, public or private organizations, government agencies, or healthcare organizations or plans—not developed or issued by an individual who is not sponsored or supported by one of these.
- Based upon a systematic literature search and review of scientific evidence published in peer-reviewed journals.
- A full text of the guideline is available in the English language.

Note. Based on information from National Guideline Clearinghouse, n.d.

Oncology Nursing Society PEP Resources Development Process

As previously described (Eaton & Tipton, 2009), PEP project teams summarize and categorize the full range of evidence for each nursing-sensitive patient outcome, or topic area. Topics areas for research and resource development have been determined through survey of select ONS membership groups (Doorenbos et al., 2008).

PEP project teams include advanced practice nurses (APNs), nurse scientists, nurse educators, and staff nurses so that a variety of expertise and perspective is provided throughout the process. PEP teams collaborate to identify the search strategy and work in pairs to review, critique, and summarize all of the intervention research studies published within at least the last five years. Once all the evidence is summarized, the teams synthesize the information for each intervention and categorize the interventions according to the ONS PEP categories of evidence using the detailed criteria for categorization as shown in Figure 1-2. The teams apply these criteria through discussion in order to achieve consensus for a category assignment. ONS members who have clinical and research experience in the topic area then peer-review all materials developed by the team.

Resources

In addition to this volume and the original book published in 2009, PEP Resources continue to be provided in open access on the ONS Web site. The types of resources and available formats continue to evolve based on input from practicing nurses to meet a variety of user preferences. A description of the PEP Resources currently available is shown in Table 1-2.

Figure 1-2. PEP Decision Rules for Summative Evaluation of Evidence

Recommended for Practice

Interventions for which effectiveness has been demonstrated by strong evidence from rigorously designed studies, meta-analyses, or systematic reviews, and for which expectation of harms is small compared with the benefits.

- Supportive evidence from at least two well-conducted randomized controlled trials that were performed at more than one institutional site and that included a sample size of at least 100 participants
- Evidence from a meta-analysis or systematic review of research studies that incorporated quality ratings in the analysis and included a total of 100 patients or more in its estimate of effect size and confidence intervals
- Recommendations from a panel of experts that derive from an explicit literature search strategy and include thorough analysis, quality rating, and synthesis of the evidence

Likely to Be Effective

Interventions for which the evidence is less well established than for those listed under Recommended for Practice.

- Supportive evidence from a single well-conducted, randomized controlled trial that included fewer than 100 patients or was conducted at one or more institutions
- Evidence from a meta-analysis or systematic review that incorporated quality ratings in the analysis and included fewer than 100 patients, or had no estimates of effect size and confidence intervals
- Evidence from a synthetic review of randomized trials that incorporated quality ratings in the analysis
- Guidelines developed largely by consensus/expert opinion rather than primarily based on the evidence and published by a panel of experts, and that are not supported by synthesis and quality rating of the evidence

Benefits Balanced With Harms

Interventions for which clinicians and patients should weigh the beneficial and harmful effects according to individual circumstances and priorities.

- Supportive evidence from one or more randomized trials, meta-analyses, or systematic reviews, but where the intervention may be associated, in certain patient populations, with adverse effects that produce or potentially produce mortality, significant morbidity, functional disability, hospitalization, or excess length of stay

Effectiveness Not Established

Interventions for which there are currently insufficient data or data of inadequate quality.

- Supportive evidence from a well-conducted case control study
- Supportive evidence from a poorly controlled or uncontrolled study
- Evidence from randomized clinical trials with one or more major or three or more minor methodologic flaws that could invalidate the results
- Evidence from nonexperimental studies with high potential for bias (such as case series with comparison to historical controls).
- Evidence from case series or case reports
- Conflicting evidence, but where the preponderance of the evidence is in support of the recommendation or meta-analysis showing a trend that did not reach statistical significance

(Continued on next page)

Figure 1-2. PEP Decision Rules for Summative Evaluation of Evidence
(Continued)

Effectiveness Unlikely

Interventions for which lack of effectiveness is less well established than for those listed under Not Recommended for Practice.
- Evidence from a single well-conducted randomized trial with at least 100 participants or conducted at more than one site and which showed no benefit for the intervention
- Evidence from a well-conducted case control study, a poorly controlled or uncontrolled study, a randomized trial with major methodologic flaws, or an observational study (e.g., case series with historical controls) that showed no benefit and a prominent and unacceptable pattern of adverse events and serious toxicities (*Common Terminology for Adverse Events* [CTCAE] grade III/IV)

Not Recommended for Practice

Interventions for which ineffectiveness or harmfulness has been demonstrated by clear evidence, or the cost or burden necessary for the intervention exceeds anticipated benefit.
- Evidence from two or more well-conducted randomized trials with at least 100 participants or conducted at more than one site and which showed no benefit for the intervention, and excessive costs or burden expected
- Evidence from a single well-conducted trial that showed a prominent and unacceptable pattern of adverse events and serious toxicities (CTCAE grade III/IV)
- Evidence from a meta-analysis or systematic review of research studies that incorporated quality ratings in the analysis and included a total of 100 patients or more in its estimate of effect size and confidence intervals with demonstrated lack of benefit or prominent and unacceptable toxicities
- Intervention discouraged from use by a panel of experts in the related subject after conducting a systematic examination, quality rating, and synthesis of the available evidence

Note. From ONS PEP (Putting Evidence Into Practice) Weight of Evidence Classification Schema: Decision Rules for Summative Evaluation of a Body of Evidence. Retrieved from http://ons.org/Research/media/ons/docs/research/outcomes/weight-of-evidence-table.pdf. Copyright by the Oncology Nursing Society. Reprinted with permission.

In 2009, the ONS Web site editorial board also developed and implemented evidence-based resources for patients based upon the PEP Resources. Information for patients is provided on the ONS patient Web site, www.thecancerjourney.org, that is evidence based and categorized for patients from five stars (most helpful) to zero stars (not recommended), to align with the standard PEP categories of evidence. These Web pages also provide a PDF version of the information that can be downloaded or printed out to provide directly to the patient.

Nursing-Sensitive Patient Outcomes and Patient-Centered Care

It is well known that EBP improves patient outcomes. Studies have shown that patients who received evidence-based nursing care experienced considerable

Table 1-2. Types of Oncology Nursing Society PEP Resources Available

Resource	Description
Print and Electronic Resources	
Putting Evidence Into Practice: Improving Oncology Patient Outcomes (book)	Summary, critique, and categorization of evidence, problem definition, incidence, assessment, and case study example for each PEP topic Available in print and electronic format Individual chapters and PEP resources available in electronic format
iPhone application	Individual topic applications available Provides PEP Resource categorized evidence summary
Web-Based Resources for Healthcare Professionals (www.ons.org/Research/PEP)	
Tables of evidence	Comprehensive summary and critique of each intervention study in PEP categorization framework
Guidelines table	Comprehensive summary and critique of published guidelines related to the topic
Systematic review/meta-analysis table	Comprehensive summary and critique of systematic reviews of and meta-analysis of interventions available for the topic area
Expert opinion table	Comprehensive summary and critique of expert opinion references regarding interventions in the topic area
Definitions table	Definitions for key terms used in the PEP resources for the topic
Quick view	One-page printable summary of interventions by PEP category
Reference list	Complete list of references used in Web-based PEP resources
Measurement summary	Review of key instruments that have been used to measure the relevant patient outcomes Provides instrument description, source, and basic psychometric properties
Web-Based Resources for Patients and Caregivers (www.thecancerjourney.org/side)	
Side effect Web pages on www.thecancerjourney.org	Provides treatment for side effects summarized and categorized from most helpful to not recommended. Information mirrors that of the professional PEP resources, stated in lay terms. Web pages provide a printable Adobe PDF document with this information that can be provided to patients

improvement in behavioral knowledge and physiologic and psychosocial outcomes compared to patients who received routine nursing care (Heater, Becker, & Olson, 1988). In order to determine the best interventions to maximize patient outcomes, nurses use different sources of knowledge such as ethical knowledge, empirical knowledge, and patient preferences (Ciliska, Pinelli, DiCenso, & Cullum, 2001). Because ONS PEP Resources identify evidence-based oncology nursing interventions, they are critical in today's healthcare environment. Nurses often do not have the time to retrieve, review, critique, summarize, and synthesize the scientific literature when caring for patients. PEP Resources address this issue by providing the compiled evidence for the practicing nurse.

Patient outcomes have generated great interest in the healthcare community since accountability has become an important expectation of the healthcare system (Pringle & Doran, 2003). Outcomes demonstrating that nurses make a difference to patients and their illness experience are necessary to show the value of nursing to health care. Nursing-sensitive patient outcomes are responsive to nursing interventions and include symptom management, physical function, performance status, quality of life, patient satisfaction, resource usage, and cost (Given & Sherwood, 2005). Patient-centered outcomes focus on healthcare outcomes that are important to the patient and include patient preference, patient satisfaction, and health-related quality of life (Oliver & Greenberg, 2009). Patient-centered outcomes are dependent on the healthcare provider's understanding of the patient's values, beliefs, and preferences. This knowledge is important in patient-centered care and EBP.

A patient-centered, evidence-based approach to care involves three steps: (a) identifying effective nursing interventions based on the best available evidence, (b) consulting with the patients to determine their preference for alternative nursing interventions, and (c) taking into account patients' preferences when providing nursing care (Sidani, Epstein, & Miranda, 2006). The patient's response to the nursing intervention is then measured. Outcomes data inform and improve nursing practice. An intervention may show effectiveness in a rigorously controlled trial, but this does not guarantee it will work just the same way in the clinical setting. Through the linking of outcomes to nursing interventions, nurses learn what is effective in the delivery of quality patient care (Ingersoll, 2005).

The most beneficial patient outcome measures are reliable, valid, appropriate to the population of interest, and sensitive to changes within and across individuals. Factors that contribute to the usefulness and accuracy of outcome measures in the clinical setting include practicality, utility, affordability, availability, and simplicity (Ingersoll, 2005). Patient self-report scales such as the numeric rating scale or visual analog scale are common outcome measures in the oncology clinical setting because they attend to all of these factors.

In selecting an outcome measure, it is important to consider all of the patient outcomes that the intervention may influence. For example, outcomes such as physical function, mood, endurance, sleep, appetite, and interpersonal interactions may improve with pain treatment and better reflect the effectiveness of analgesic therapy than self-reported pain intensity ratings in older adults with cancer (Miaskowski, 2010). Thus, it is essential to consider measuring multiple patient outcomes when evaluating nursing care effectiveness in specific patient populations.

Implementation

Since the PEP resources were initially introduced, the emphasis has been on getting the materials into the bedside or chairside nurse's hands through print or electronic format. Accessibility continues to be a priority, but an additional area of focus is that of translation of the evidence that is now summarized and available into direct nursing practice. In examining the area of EBP implementation or translation into practice, it is useful to explore three main areas: basic types of implementation in practice, current evidence about what works for implementation, and the experiences of ONS members in using PEP resources to facilitate practice change.

Basic Types of Implementation

In looking at the issue of implementing EBP, it is important to recognize the difference between the individual nurse making use of the evidence in his or her own personal practice and implementing EBP among a group of nurses who work together to provide care.

For nurses who work independently and those who incorporate evidence into personal care approaches, translation of evidence into practice is a relatively straightforward process of (a) assessing the patients' needs, (b) identifying the PEP resources that address those patient needs, (c) selecting those interventions that have both the highest category of evidence and are acceptable and helpful to the individual patient, (d) incorporating those interventions into the plan of care and execution of that plan, and (e) evaluating the effects of the intervention. The evidence is used throughout the nursing process with individuals or cohorts of patients. Tips for using the PEP resources are posted on the ONS Web site (www.ons.org/Research/PEP).

Implementing PEP resources among a multidisciplinary group or a team of nurses involves additional actions and skills in order to create practice change. This aspect of implementation is an area of current interest. Many terms have been applied to describe these processes, including *implementation science*, *improvement science*, *translation science*, *knowledge transfer*, and *knowledge translation*. Although these labels differ and the concepts they incorporate may also differ, their aim is much the same: bringing the evidence to life in the practice of nursing and other disciplines. Just as the use of the evidence is essential to improve patient care quality, the use of the evidence to implement practice change is helpful to the EBP change efforts, no matter what terminology is used or model is applied.

Current Evidence About What Works to Implement Evidence-Based Practice

In a broad review of models, strategies, and measurement approaches, Sudsawad (2007) summarized some of the evidence regarding effectiveness of implementation strategies from studies and systematic reviews. Titler (2008) also provided an overview of the evidence about what is known regarding implementing evidence-based practices. It is clear that the process of implementing EBP is an extremely complex one, given the diverse nature of practice, practitioners, and the settings in which changes occur. Evidence is limited about what specific actions work best in implementing EBP, and it is difficult to draw conclusions about how to best promote evidence usage that can be generalized to a wide variety of settings and circumstances. However, these reviews do point to some consistent themes and findings that can be incorporated into implementation planning, including the following.

- Implementation combining use of more than one strategy appears to be essential to promote the use of evidence.
- Passive provision of evidence to potential end users generally is not effective. Individuals whose practice is to be modified need to be actively engaged in the change process.

Strategies that were found to be consistently effective or to a high degree in studies included

- Education and educational outreach, particularly interactive education
- Use of reminders and practice cues
- Marketing the practice change
- Auditing and feedback.

Tailored interventions designed to meet individualized organizational assessment of the gap between evidence and practice and overcome specific barriers to change is another approach to facilitate evidence translation (Titler, 2008). The tailored approach involves organizational assessment to identify areas of strength and opportunities for improvement in terms of factors that influence the gap between evidence and practice in that particular setting.

Oncology Nursing Society Members' Experiences in Use and Implementation of PEP Resources and Evidence-Based Practice

Additional sources of evidence and creative ideas about how to implement the use of evidence into practice are the responses, experiences, and stories of others who have taken these actions. ONS conducted three surveys in 2007 and 2008, including 975 Society members. One sample was obtained from conference attendees who ordered PEP cards, one was a convenience sample of 2008 ONS Congress attendees, and the third was a random sample of 405 nurses who worked in ambulatory settings in 2008. Data were also obtained from an additional 41 members via focus groups and interviews regarding PEP resources and resource use.

Survey results about the types of use of PEP resources across all survey groups are presented in Table 1-3. As shown here, the most frequently reported use was nurse and caregiver education, reported by 56% of survey participants. Other uses included discussion with other nurses (49.9%); use for patient care and care planning (45.5%); patient education (39.4%); discussions among the healthcare team, either formally through committees or informally as in physician rounds (27%); and incorporation of the evidence into policy, procedure, guidelines, and standing physician orders (10.6%). Consolidation of open-ended comments in these surveys and findings from focus groups and interviews yielded the following common implementation strategies used by members whose experiences showed they were effective.

- Incorporation into nursing documentation
- Policy and standards of practice development
- Incorporation of evidence into standing physician orders
- Individual patient-focused discussion with the physician
- Incorporation of use into clinical ladder requirements and expectations
- Education of nurses, other caregivers, and other professional staff
- Journal clubs
- Discussion of and reference to PEP resources in nursing report
- Placement of the PEP Web page link on the organization's intranet

One of the key points that many respondents made in interviews was that in working toward EBP, it is important for nurses to embrace the idea that the use of evidence is key to providing quality patient care. Use of evidence is not for the sake of itself—the purpose is quality patient care and better patient outcomes.

Educating nurses and other disciplines can be performed through orientation, in-services, conferences, skills laboratories, competency development, and the ONS Chemotherapy and Biotherapy Course. Other opportunities include journal clubs, research roundtables, shared governance meetings, nursing councils, other formal organization groups and committees, and staff meetings (Gurzick & Kesten, 2010; Harne-Britner & Schafer, 2009; Warren & Thompson, 2010). Education is one main technique to increase knowledge and awareness, but as Titler (2009) pointed out, "education alone is never enough to change practice . . . simply improving knowledge does not necessarily improve practice" (p. 11).

In addition to such educational approaches, some clinical nurse specialists have discussed using the PEP materials on bulletin boards, one on one in nursing rounds, and

Table 1-3. Consolidated Oncology Nursing Society Member Survey Results Regarding Types of PEP Resource Used (N = 975 in three member surveys, 2007–2008)		
Type of Use	**Percent of Total**	**Range Across Surveys**
Nurse and caregiver education	56%	N/A*
Inform and discuss with other nurses	49.9%	30%–64%
Patient care and care planning	45.5%	16.4%–74%
Patient education	39.4%	20.5%–62%
Discussion in the healthcare team • In-team meetings • MD rounds • Committees	27%	13.5%–54%
Incorporate into policy, procedure, guidelines, or standing physician orders	10.6%	N/A*
*This survey selection item was only available in one survey of ambulatory nurses (n = 405).		

through staff huddles. Integration into electronic medical records has also begun in some settings. This approach is in its infancy for most organizations and would ultimately be an extremely valuable way to provide reminders, as well as the format for documentation. Such documentation could enable more automated data collection for quality auditing.

Next Steps in the Oncology Nursing Society PEP Journey

ONS has a strong commitment to EBP and the continued provision of resources for nurses to make it easier for them to use the best evidence in their practices. Within the PEP program, goals include making the evidence available at the point of care and the continued development of resources that the nurses say they need. The next steps in the PEP program and EBP are

- Development and implementation of processes to achieve more current updating of resources
- Continued development of additional resource formats and structure to meet nurses' varied preferences for access and use
- Increased collaboration and usage by other nursing and professional groups. Although the ONS PEP resources are oncology focused, the materials have relevance for some other patient types and other disciplines that work with these patients.
- Programs to facilitate the process of practice change.

Nurses are in key positions to become change agents, are quite capable of applying the evidence, and understand the barriers and facilitators of improvement (Doran & Sidani, 2007; Fineout-Overholt, Williamson, Kent, & Hutchinson, 2010; Kent, Hutchinson, & Fineout-Overholt, 2009; Profetto-McGrath, Negrin, Hugo, & Smith, 2010). The PEP resources provide one bridge between evidence and practice by putting the evidence at the fingertips of those who can use it. These resources are designed to improve patient outcomes by providing effective evidence-based nursing interventions. The measurement of both patient-centered and nursing-sensitive outcomes is critical to this process. Outcomes data inform nursing practice and enable continuous improvement in the quality of care.

References

Ciliska, D.K., Pinelli, J., DiCenso, A., & Cullum, N. (2001). Resources to enhance evidence-based nursing practice. *AACN Clinical Issues, 12,* 520–528.

Doorenbos, A.Z., Berger, A.M., Brohard-Holbert, C., Eaton, L., Kozachik, S., LoBiondo-Wood, G., … Varricchio, C. (2008). Oncology Nursing Society Putting Evidence Into Practice Resources: Where are we now and what is next? *Clinical Journal of Oncology Nursing, 12,* 965–970. doi:10.1188/08.CJON.965-970

Doran, D.M., & Sidani, S. (2007). Outcomes-focused knowledge translation: A framework for knowledge translation and patient outcomes improvement. *Worldviews on Evidence-Based Nursing, 4,* 3–13. doi:10.1111/j.1741-6787.2007.00073.x

Eaton, L.H., & Tipton, J.M. (Eds.). (2009). *Putting evidence into practice: Improving oncology patient outcomes.* Pittsburgh, PA: Oncology Nursing Society.

Fineout-Overholt, E., Williamson, K.M., Kent, B., & Hutchinson, A.M. (2010). Teaching EBP: Strategies for achieving sustainable organizational change toward evidence-based practice. *Worldviews on Evidence-Based Nursing, 7,* 51–53. doi:10.1111/j.1741-6787.2010.00185.x

Given, B.A., & Sherwood, P.R. (2005). Nursing-sensitive patient outcomes—A white paper. *Oncology Nursing Forum, 32,* 773–784. doi:10.1188/04.ONF.773-784

Gurzick, M., & Kesten, K.S. (2010). The impact of clinical nurse specialists on clinical pathways in the application of evidence-based practice. *Journal of Professional Nursing, 26,* 42–48. doi:10.1016/j.profnurs.2009.04.003

Harne-Britner, S., & Schafer, D.J. (2009). Clinical nurse specialists driving research and practice through research roundtables. *Clinical Nurse Specialist, 23,* 305–308. doi:10.1097/NUR.0b013e3181bc30c9

Heater, B.S., Becker, A.M., & Olson, R.K. (1988). Nursing interventions and patient outcomes: A meta-analysis of studies. *Nursing Research, 37,* 303–307.

Ingersoll, G.L. (2005). Generating evidence through outcomes management. In B.M. Melnyk & E. Fineout-Overholt (Eds.), *Evidence-based practice in nursing and healthcare: A guide to best practice* (pp. 299–332). Philadelphia, PA: Lippincott Williams & Wilkins.

Kent, B., Hutchinson, A.M., & Fineout-Overholt, E. (2009). Getting evidence into practice: Understanding knowledge translation to achieve practice change. *Worldviews on Evidence-Based Nursing, 6,* 183–185. doi:10.1111/j.1741-6787.2009.00165.x

Miaskowski, C. (2010). Outcome measures to evaluate the effectiveness of pain management in older adults with cancer. *Oncology Nursing Forum, 37*(Suppl.), 27–32. doi:10.1188/10.ONF.S1.27-32

National Guideline Clearinghouse. (n.d.). Inclusion criteria. Retrieved from http://guidelines.gov/about/inclusion-criteria.aspx

Oliver, A., & Greenberg, C.C. (2009). Measuring outcomes in oncology treatment: The importance of patient-centered outcomes. *Surgical Clinics of North America, 89,* 17–25. doi:10.1016/j.suc.2008.09.015

Oncology Nursing Society Survivorship Think Tank. (2009, April 9). *ONS cancer survivorship initiatives roadmap.* Unpublished manuscript, Oncology Nursing Society, Pittsburgh, PA.

Pringle, D., & Doran, D.M. (2003). Patient outcomes as an accountability. In D. Doran (Ed.), *Nursing sensitive outcomes: State of the science* (pp. 1–26). Sudbury, MA: Jones and Bartlett.

Profetto-McGrath, J., Negrin, K.A., Hugo, K., & Smith, K.B. (2010). Clinical nurse specialists' approaches in selecting and using evidence to improve practice. *Worldviews on Evidence-Based Nursing, 7,* 36–50. doi:10.1111/j.1741-6787.2009.00164.x

Sidani, S., Epstein, D., & Miranda, J. (2006). Eliciting patient treatment preferences: A strategy to integrate evidence-based and patient centered care. *Worldviews on Evidence-Based Nursing, 3,* 116–123. doi:10.1111/j.1741-6787.2006.00060.x

Sudsawad, P. (2007). *Knowledge translation: Introduction to models, strategies, and measures.* Retrieved from http://www.ncddr.org/kt/products/ktintro

Titler, M.G. (2008). The evidence for evidence-based practice implementation. In R. Hughes (Ed.), *Patient safety and quality: An evidence-based handbook for nurses.* Retrieved from http://www.ncbi.nlm.nih.gov/bookshelf/br.fcgi?book=nursehb&part=ch7

Warren, J.J., & Thompson, T.L. (2010). Quality and safety education for the nurses competencies for the clinical nurse specialist. *Clinical Nurse Specialist, 24,* 187–188. doi:10.1097/NUR.0b013c3181c653f6

CHAPTER **2**

Cognitive Impairment

Editor, Deborah Hutchinson Allen, MSN, CNS, FNP-BC, AOCNP®

Problem

Cognitive function is a multidimensional concept that describes the domains resulting from healthy brain performance, namely attention and concentration, executive function, information processing speed, language, visuospatial skill, psychomotor ability, learning, and memory (Jansen, Miaskowski, Dodd, Dowling, & Kramer, 2005b). Cognitive impairment can be defined as a decline in function in either one or multiple domains of cognitive function. Cognitive impairment is a distressing symptom that can occur as a direct result of cancer or its treatment and may persist after the treatment has been completed.

Incidence

The incidence of this symptom may vary depending on the type of cancer, type of treatment, patient's time since diagnosis, and how cognitive impairment is defined and measured. Initial research regarding cognitive impairment in patients with cancer focused on patients with brain tumors. In this population, cognitive impairment was reported in 50%–80% of patients with brain tumors at the time of diagnosis (Tucha, Smely, Preier, & Lange, 2000), suggesting that deficits are mainly the result of the tumor itself (Taphoorn, 2009). Recently, evidence suggests that cognitive impairment is also present in other populations prior to the initiation of treatment. Longitudinal studies that included neuropsychological testing prior to treatment demonstrated preexisting cognitive impairment in 11%–35% of patients with breast cancer (Ahles et al., 2007; Hermelink et al., 2007; Hurria et al., 2006; Jansen, Dodd, Miaskowski, Dowling, & Kramer, 2008; Wefel, Lenzi, Theriault, Davis, & Meyers, 2004), 70%–80% of patients with lung cancer (Meyers, Byrne, & Komaki, 1995), and 40% of patients with acute myeloid leukemia (Meyers, Albitar, & Este, 2005).

Further research has found that clinically significant cognitive impairment may continue well after treatment has been completed (Von Ah, Russell, Storniolo, & Carpenter, 2009). Several meta-analyses (Anderson-Hanley, Sherman, Riggs,

15

Agocha, & Compas, 2003; Falleti, Sanfilippo, Maruff, Weih, & Phillips, 2005; Jansen, Miaskowski, Dodd, Dowling, & Kramer, 2005a; Stewart, Bielajew, Collins, Parkinson, & Tomiak, 2006) documented that treatment-related cognitive impairments occur in cancer survivors, with the majority reporting deficits in memory, speed of processing, and executive and psychomotor functioning. Although cross-sectional studies have reported cognitive impairment in 15%–75% of adult solid tumor survivors who received chemotherapy, more recent longitudinal studies suggest that this number is closer to 20%–30% of cancer survivors with lingering cancer- or cancer treatment–related cognitive impairments (Vardy, Wefel, Ahles, Tannock, & Schagen, 2007; Von Ah, Harvison, et al., 2009). Given the sheer numbers of cancer survivors and significant impact cognitive impairment can have on quality of life (Mehnert et al., 2007; Von Ah, Russell, et al., 2009), cognitive impairment is an important symptom to address.

Prevention

Currently, evidence-based preventive measures for cancer- and cancer treatment–related cognitive impairment do not exist. It is hoped that once more is understood about the underlying physiologic mechanisms associated with this problem that interventions can be developed and tested to prevent and treat cognitive impairments.

Survivorship

Changes in cognitive function as a result of the cancer or treatment can be distressing and life impacting for many cancer survivors. Little is known about the actual prevalence, duration, and trajectory of cognitive impairments in patients with cancer. However, cancer survivors report that cognitive problems exist, and this impairment can dramatically affect their overall quality of life (Ahles & Saykin, 2001; Cull et al., 1996; Mehnert et al., 2007; Reid-Arndt, 2006; Von Ah, Russell, et al., 2009).

In a recent survey of 471 cancer survivors, 62% stated that cognitive problems were disruptive to their functioning and relationships both at home and at work (Hede, 2008). At work, cancer survivors with cognitive impairment expressed feelings of being overwhelmed and reported difficulties with making decisions and multitasking, and others reported a lack of self-confidence in their overall work performance (Calvio, Peugeot, Bruns, Todd, & Feuerstein, 2010; Munir, Burrows, Yarker, Kalawsky, & Bains, 2010). Researchers have also documented that cancer survivors with problems with attention experience more depressive symptoms, lower well-being, poorer physical functioning, and greater fatigue (Von Ah, Russell, et al., 2009), and survivors with problems with their memory experience poorer physical and emotional functioning up to five years after chemotherapy (Mehnert et al., 2007). Although cognitive impairments may appear subtle, they can significantly affect the survivors' quality of life as well as their ability to function in occupational, social, and daily life activities (Fitch, Armstrong, & Tsang, 2008).

A frequent frustration expressed by survivors is the lack of information provided by medical professionals regarding cancer- and cancer treatment–related cognitive impairments (Boykoff, Moieni, & Subramanian, 2009; Fitch et al., 2008). Despite limitations in understanding this phenomenon, acknowledgment and validation of patient reports is essential. Patients should be informed that cognitive changes are possible side effects of cancer and cancer-related treatment, and although little is known, studies are ongoing.

Assessment

Recognizing changes in cognitive function in patients with cancer is important throughout the trajectory of the cancer experience. Survivors have reported that subtle declines in memory, concentration, and executive functioning occur during the acute phase of treatment and frequently persist after treatment is completed. Although numerous neuropsychological tests exist, they require special training to administer. Furthermore, limited information is available on specificity and sensitivity in regard to measuring cancer- and treatment-related cognitive changes (Jansen, Miaskowski, Dodd, & Dowling, 2007). However, a detailed assessment of the patient's reports of cognitive problems (e.g., forgetfulness; difficulty with memory, word finding, or multitasking) as well as suspected contributing factors can be useful in determining other potentially treatable causes (see Figure 2-1). Clinicians should pay close attention to the patient's reports of cognitive changes and consider assessment with a subjective instrument. Persistent or worsening symptoms may warrant a referral to a neuropsychologist for a comprehensive focused cognitive assessment.

Assessing patients for cognitive impairment is difficult because of the lack of clinically useful instrument tools. Currently, this relies on subjective self-report surveys or objective clinician-administered tests (see Table 2-1). Subjective tools require the patient or caregiver to report cognitive functioning concerns; however, not all patients will be forthcoming about their concerns because of fear or embarrassment. In contrast, trained neuropsychology clinicians administer objective tools, and each test can identify specific cognitive domains that may be impaired. Objective neuropsychological testing is considered the preferred method of identifying cognitive impairment in other patient populations (e.g., stroke, head injury, Alzheimer disease); however, concerns have been raised as to whether they fully capture the more subtle cognitive impairment noted in patients with cancer. One objective measure that is used widely in the clinical setting to screen for global cognitive impairment is the Mini-Mental State Examination (MMSE). This objective measure should be used with caution because recent research has found that it disproportionately identifies individuals with lower intelligence or education as impaired while failing to identify impairment in well-educated individuals. Additionally, even when trained professionals administer the test, the MMSE is not sensitive enough to detect subtle cognitive changes that may occur in patients with cancer (Meyers & Wefel, 2003). To date, no subjective or objective tools are recommended to be routinely administered in the clinical situation to easily identify cognitive impairments. Instead, nurse clinicians are encouraged to consider using a combination of patient reports of cognitive concerns and clinical assessment of difficulty with routine functioning (e.g., forgetting appointment times, difficulty remembering medication schedules) and referring patients when warranted to neuropsychologists for further evaluation.

Figure 2-1. Cognitive Assessment Guide		
Cancer History	**Specific Information (Including Dates) or Not Applicable (NA)**	
Cancer diagnosis/stage		
Surgery		
Radiation therapy		
Chemotherapy		
Hormonal therapy		
Immunotherapy		
Potential Contributing Factors	**Yes**	**No**
Anemia		
Cardiovascular disease		
Depression		
Diabetes mellitus		
Drug or alcohol abuse		
Fatigue		
Head injury		
Insomnia/sleep disturbance		
Medication (i.e., analgesics, antidepressants, antiepileptics, anxiolytics, antipsychotics, immunosuppressants, steroids)		
Neurologic conditions (e.g., stroke, Alzheimer disease)		
Nutritional deficiencies		
Psychiatric illnesses		
Cognitive Changes (patient reports difficulty with):	**Yes**	**No**
Memory		
Word finding		
Concentration/focus		
Executive functioning/goal-directed behaviors		
Other (state):		

Table 2-1. Sample of Subjective Instruments Used to Measure Cognitive Function					
Name of Tool	**Number of Items**	**Domains**	**Reliability and Validity**	**Populations**	**Clinical Utility**
Attentional Function Index	13	Attention, executive function, working memory	Adequate reliability and validity established	Breast and lung cancers	Short and easy to administer
Cognitive Failures Questionnaire	25	Perception, memory, attention	Adequate reliability	Breast cancer, gliomas	Easy to administer
Functional Assessment of Cancer Therapy–Cognitive	50	Mental acuity, concentration, verbal and nonverbal memory, verbal fluency	Adequate reliability and validity	Various cancer types, including breast, multiple myeloma, non-Hodgkin lymphoma, and prostate	Somewhat long for clinical use but easy to administer and interpret
Patient's Assessment of Own Functioning	33	Memory, executive function, language and communication, sensory-perceptual and motor skills	Sufficient reliability and validity established	Breast cancer	Somewhat long for clinical use but easy to administer
Perception of Cognition Questionnaire	7	Attention and concentration, executive function, memory, language	Limited reliability and validity	Breast cancer	Easy to use and designed to assess changes over time

References

Ahles, T.A., & Saykin, A.J. (2001). Cognitive effects of standard-dose chemotherapy in patients with cancer. *Cancer Investigation, 19,* 812–820.

Ahles, T.A., Saykin, A.J., McDonald, B.C., Furstenberg, C.T., Cole, B.F., Hanscom, B.S., … Kaufman, P.A. (2007). Cognitive function in breast cancer patients prior to adjuvant treatment. *Cancer Research and Treatment, 110,* 143–152. doi:10.1007/s10549-007-9686-5

Anderson-Hanley, C., Sherman, M.L., Riggs, R., Agocha, V.B., & Compas, B.E. (2003). Neuropsychological effects of treatments for adults with cancer: A meta-analysis and review of the literature. *Journal of the International Neuropsychological Society, 9,* 967–982. doi:10.1017/S1355617703970019

Boykoff, N., Moieni, M., & Subramanian, S.K. (2009). Confronting chemo brain: An in-depth look at survivors' reports of impact on work, social networks, and health care response. *Journal of Cancer Survivorship, 3,* 223–232. doi:10.1007/s11764-009-0098-x

Calvio, L., Peugeot, M., Bruns, G.L., Todd, B.L., & Feuerstein, M. (2010). Measures of cognitive function and work in occupationally active breast cancer survivors. *Journal of Occupational and Environmental Medicine, 52,* 219–227. doi:10.1097/JOM.0b013e3181d0bef7

Cull, A., Hay, C., Love, S.B., Mackie, M., Smets, E., & Stewart, M. (1996). What do cancer patients mean when they complain of concentration and memory problems? *British Journal of Cancer, 74,* 1674–1679. Retrieved from http://www.ncbi.nlm.nih.gov/pmc/articles/PMC2074867/?tool=pubmed

Falleti, M.G., Sanfilippo, A., Maruff, P., Weih, L., & Phillips, K.A. (2005). The nature and severity of cognitive impairment associated with adjuvant chemotherapy in women with breast cancer: A meta-analysis of the current literature. *Brain and Cognition, 59,* 60–70. doi:10.1016/j.bandc.2005.05.001

Fitch, M.I., Armstrong, J., & Tsang, S. (2008). Patients' experiences with cognitive changes after chemotherapy. *Canadian Oncology Nursing Journal, 18,* 180–192.

Hede, K. (2008). Chemobrain is real but may need new name. *Journal of the National Cancer Institute, 100,* 162–163, 169. doi:10.1093/jnci/djn007

Hermelink, K., Untch, M., Lux, M.P., Kreienberg, R., Beck, T., Bauerfeind, I., & Münzel, K. (2007). Cognitive function during neoadjuvant chemotherapy for breast cancer: Results of a prospective, multicenter, longitudinal study. *Cancer, 109,* 1905–1913. doi:10.1002/cncr.22610

Hurria, A., Rosen, C., Hudis, C., Zuckerman, E., Panageas, K.S., Lachs, M.S., … Holland, J. (2006). Cognitive function of older patients receiving adjuvant chemotherapy for breast cancer: A pilot prospective longitudinal study. *Journal of the American Geriatrics Society, 54,* 926–931. doi:10.1111/j.1532-5415.2006.00732.x

Jansen, C.E., Dodd, M.J., Miaskowski, C.A., Dowling, G.A., & Kramer, J. (2008). Preliminary results of a longitudinal study of changes in cognitive function in breast cancer patients undergoing chemotherapy with doxorubicin and cyclophosphamide. *Psycho-Oncology, 17,* 1189–1195. doi:10.1002/pon.1342

Jansen, C.E., Miaskowski, C.A., Dodd, M.J., & Dowling, G.A. (2007). A meta-analysis of the sensitivity of various neuropsychological tests used to detect chemotherapy-induced cognitive impairment in patients with breast cancer. *Oncology Nursing Forum, 34,* 997–1005. doi:10.1188/07.ONF.997-1005

Jansen, C.E., Miaskowski, C.A., Dodd, M.J., Dowling, G.A., & Kramer, J. (2005a). A meta-analysis of studies of the effects of cancer chemotherapy on various domains of cognitive function. *Cancer, 104,* 2222–2233. doi:10.1002/cncr.21469

Jansen, C.E., Miaskowski, C.A., Dodd, M.J., Dowling, G.A., & Kramer, J. (2005b). Potential mechanisms for chemotherapy-induced impairments in cognitive function. *Oncology Nursing Forum, 32,* 1151–1163.

Mehnert, A., Scherwath, A., Schirmer, L., Schleimer, B., Petersen, C., Schulz-Kindermann, F., … Koch, U. (2007). The association between neuropsychological impairment, self-perceived cognitive deficits, fatigue and health related quality of life in breast cancer survivors following standard adjuvant versus high-dose chemotherapy. *Patient Education and Counseling, 66,* 108–118. doi:10.1016/j.pec.2006.11.005

Meyers, C.A., Albitar, M., & Este, E. (2005). Cognitive impairment, fatigue, and cytokine levels in patients with acute myelogenous leukemia or myelodysplastic syndrome. *Cancer, 104,* 788–793. doi:10.1002/cncr.21234

Meyers, C.A., Byrne, K.S., & Komaki, R. (1995). Cognitive deficits in patients with small cell lung cancer before and after chemotherapy. *Lung Cancer, 12,* 231–235. doi:10.1016/0169-5002(95)00446-8

Meyers, C.A., & Wefel, J.S. (2003). The use of the Mini-Mental State Examination to assess cognitive functioning in cancer trials: No ifs, ands, buts, or sensitivity. *Journal of Clinical Oncology, 21,* 3557–3558. doi:10.1200/JCO.2003.07.080

Munir, F., Burrows, J., Yarker, J., Kalawsky, K., & Bains, M. (2010). Women's perceptions of chemotherapy-induced cognitive side affects on work ability: A focus group study. *Journal of Clinical Nursing, 19*, 1362–1370. doi:10.1111/j.1365-2702.2009.03006.x

Reid-Arndt, S.A. (2006). The potential for neuropsychology to inform functional outcomes research with breast cancer survivors. *NeuroRehabilitation, 21*, 51–64.

Stewart, A., Bielajew, C., Collins, B., Parkinson, M., & Tomiak, E. (2006). A meta-analysis of the neuropsychological effects of adjuvant chemotherapy treatment in women treated for breast cancer. *Clinical Neuropsychologist, 20*, 76–89. doi:10.1080/138540491005875

Taphoorn, M.J.B. (2009). Neurocognitive effects of radiotherapy. In R. Govindan (Ed.), *American Society of Clinical Oncology 2009 educational book* (pp. 90–93). Alexandria, VA: American Society of Clinical Oncology.

Tucha, O., Smely, C., Preier, M., & Lange, K.W. (2000). Cognitive deficits before treatment among patients with brain tumors. *Neurosurgery, 47*, 324–333.

Vardy, J., Wefel, J.S., Ahles, T., Tannock, I.F., & Schagen, S.B. (2007). Cancer and cancer-therapy related cognitive dysfunction: An international perspective from the Venice cognitive workshop. *Annals of Oncology, 19*, 623–629. doi:10.1093/annonc/mdm500

Von Ah, D., Harvison, K.W., Monahan, P.O., Moser, L.R., Zhao, Q., Carpenter, J.S., ... Unverzagt, F.W. (2009). Cognitive function in breast cancer survivors compared to healthy age- and education-matched women. *Clinical Neuropsychologist, 23*, 661–674. doi:10.1080/13854040802541439

Von Ah, D., Russell, K., Storniolo, A.M., & Carpenter, J.S. (2009). Cognitive dysfunction and its relationship to quality of life in breast cancer survivors. *Oncology Nursing Forum, 36*, 326–334. doi:10.1188/09.ONF.326-334

Wefel, J.S., Lenzi, R., Theriault, R.L., Davis, R.N., & Meyers, C.A. (2004). The cognitive sequelae of standard-dose adjuvant chemotherapy in women with breast carcinoma: Results of a prospective, randomized, longitudinal trial. *Cancer, 100*, 2292–2299. doi:10.1002/cncr.20272

Case Study

D.F. is a married 49-year-old woman with two children (16 and 18 years old) and works as an investment banker for a multinational company. She has a master's degree in finance and commands respect in the industry. Five years ago she was diagnosed with stage 2B breast cancer (2.1 cm, 1 positive node, estrogen receptor/progesterone receptor positive, HER2 negative). Treatment consisted of a lumpectomy, initial chemotherapy of AC (doxorubicin 60 mg/m^2 and cyclophosphamide 600 mg/m^2 every 21 days) for four cycles, followed by T (paclitaxel 225 mg/m^2) for an additional four cycles. Although she was able to work through treatment, her treatment course was complicated by neutropenia, fatigue, and nausea and vomiting. Her survivorship has been complicated by chronic peripheral neuropathy of her feet.

On arrival to the Survivorship Clinic, she completed several self-assessment forms that enabled the clinicians to gain a general understanding of her current health, health promotion activities, persistent issues related to her treatment or survival, and any other fears or concerns. The oncology clinical nurse specialist (CNS) identified several key issues from the surveys that required further discussion. These included chronic neuropathy, fatigue, and possibly depression. The CNS reviewed D.F.'s current medication regimen, which consisted of 5 mg zolpidem at bedtime as needed, 1,000 mg calcium twice a day, and atorvastatin 10 mg daily for hypercholesterolemia.

During the evaluation, D.F. indicated that she was frustrated by persistent symptoms and that she "wanted to be the way [she] was." While describing her current abilities to function at work and social activities, she stated that she had problems with her memory and concentration, specifically "not being as mentally sharp as [she] used to be." While crying, she indicated that she had not shared this fear with anyone and that it was leading to considerable strain in her personal and professional relationships. Furthermore, D.F. reported problems in memory, concentration, multitasking, word finding, and comprehension. She recounted several incidents to highlight her "chemo brain" as she half-jokingly referred to her cognitive impairment. The CNS acknowledged how difficult it must have been for her to reveal these cognitive issues. She offered the patient a referral to a neuropsychologist for a detailed evaluation. In addition, the CNS explained that they could review the Oncology Nursing Society's (ONS's) evidence-based practice guidelines for any recommendations of specific interventions for cognitive impairment. She explained that these guidelines assist clinicians in reviewing interventions based on scientific evidence of effectiveness.

Together, they reviewed the ONS Putting Evidence Into Practice (PEP) information on cognitive impairment. They checked her current medications and noted that they did not have associated side effects for cognitive changes. They saw that although methylphenidate and other stimulant medications such as modafinil and donepezil have been studied, their effectiveness has not been established. The patient was relieved because she was reluctant to take more medications. She asked if any nonpharmacologic interventions might help, and the CNS stated that although nonpharmacologic interventions have been studied, not enough information was available to prove their effectiveness at that time. D.F. said she was "willing to try anything to get better." The CNS discussed the interventions to assist in the management of difficulties in thinking and perception, such as puzzles, use of day planners, and written reminders. Based on her assessment of potential contributing factors, the CNS also mentioned that fatigue can play a role in cognitive impairment; they took a few minutes to evaluate the ONS PEP resource on fatigue to see if any information was available that D.F. would be willing to try. Reviewing the evidence, D.F. agreed to an exercise program, which was the only intervention in the *Recommend for Practice* category for fatigue management.

Three months later, the patient was seen for a follow-up appointment. The CNS noticed that she exhibited an improvement in the symptom surveys for her cognitive function and fatigue. D.F. was exercising regularly and was sleeping without need for zolpidem. She talked with her husband regarding her concerns about cognitive issues and found him to be supportive. She said she has an improved quality of life and a better outlook. She attributed all of this to being honest about her cognitive issues in the first place—something she realized many survivors are afraid to do. The CNS thanked D.F. for her honesty and recognized that she needs to incorporate questions about cognitive functioning into every patient's screening.

Cognitive Impairment

AUTHORS
Deborah Hutchinson Allen, MSN, CNS, FNP-BC, AOCNP®, Diane Von Ah, PhD, RN,
Catherine Jansen, PhD, RN, CNS, OCN®, Rosalina M. Schiavone, RN, BSN, OCN®,
Phyllis Gagnon, RN, BSN, OCN®, Jennifer Wulff, RN, MN, ARNP, AOCNP®, and
Rachel Behrendt, DNP, MSN, APN-C, AOCNS®
LIBRARIAN: Mark Vrabel, MLS, AHIP, ELS
ONS STAFF: Margaret Irwin, PhD, RN, MN

What interventions are effective in managing cognitive impairment in people with cancer?

Recommended for Practice

Interventions for which effectiveness has been demonstrated by strong evidence from rigorously conducted studies, meta-analyses, or systematic reviews and for which expectation of harms is small compared with the benefits

No interventions are recommended as of February 2010.

Likely to Be Effective

Interventions for which effectiveness has been demonstrated by supportive evidence from a single rigorously conducted controlled trial, consistent supportive evidence from well-designed controlled trials using small samples, or guidelines developed from evidence and supported by expert opinion

There are no interventions as of February 2010.

Benefits Balanced With Harms

Interventions for which clinicians and patients should weigh the beneficial and harmful effects according to individual circumstances and priorities

There are no interventions as of February 2010.

Effectiveness Not Established

Interventions for which insufficient or conflicting data or data of inadequate quality currently exist, with no clear indication of harm

MEDICATIONS/PHARMACEUTICAL INTERVENTIONS

Methylphenidate
Pharmacologic interventions have focused predominately on testing the efficacy of the psychostimulant methylphenidate to address cognitive impairment in patients with cancer (Bruera,

Miller, Macmillan, & Kuehn, 1992; Butler et al., 2007; Gagnon, Low, & Schreier, 2005; Lower et al., 2009; Mar Fan et al., 2008; Meyers, Weitzner, Valentine, & Levin, 1998). Seven studies (Bruera et al., 1992; Butler et al., 2007; Gagnon et al., 2005; Lower et al., 2009; Mar Fan et al., 2008; Meyers et al., 1999; Schwartz, Thompson, & Masood, 2002) were found that tested the use of methylphenidate either alone or in combination with exercise (Schwartz et al., 2002) to treat cognitive impairment in adults with cancer. Although initial studies reported methylphenidate improved cognitive performance (increased alertness) in patients with advanced cancer (Bruera et al., 1992; Gagnon et al., 2005; Meyers et al., 1998), three recent randomized controlled trials failed to demonstrate significant effects of methylphenidate on cognitive functioning (Butler et al., 2007; Lower et al., 2009; Mar Fan et al., 2008). In fact, two of the three studies failed to recruit an adequate number of participants with cancer (Butler et al., 2007; Mar Fan et al., 2008), which may indicate that patients with cancer are not interested in taking these additional medications. Additional research is needed regarding the use of methylphenidate for cognitive functioning in patients with cancer.

Other Stimulant Medications

Researchers have also explored the use of other psychostimulant medications. Five studies were found that tested either modafinil (Blackhall, Petroni, Shu, Baum, & Farace, 2009; Kohli et al., 2009; Lundorff, Jønsson, & Sjøgren, 2009) or donepezil (Jatoi et al., 2005; Shaw et al., 2006). One of the studies examining donepezil also examined vitamin E (Jatoi et al., 2005). The results of these studies are equivocal and require further replication. The results are reported below.

Donepezil: Two studies have examined the effect of donepezil on cognitive function in adult patients with cancer (Jatoi et al., 2005; Shaw et al., 2006), one of which also simultaneously examined vitamin E (Jatoi et al., 2005). Shaw and colleagues (2006) conducted a one-arm trial of donepezil on cognitive functioning in patients with brain tumors who were receiving irradiation. This study reported some improvements in cognitive functioning, but the results may have been confounded because of simultaneous improvements in tumor size, resolution of radiation-induced fatigue, or repair and recovery from radiation-induced brain damage. Jatoi and colleagues (2005) conducted a randomized, controlled, double-blind, placebo-controlled trial and failed to find a significant effect of donepezil and vitamin E on cognitive functioning. However, this study was stopped prematurely because of failure to recruit participants (only nine subjects enrolled). This failure to recruit subjects into the study may reflect that patients with cancer were unwilling to take one or both of these medications. Research exploring donepezil use is limited by study designs (no randomized controlled trials) and small samples sizes and thus would require further research to establish effectiveness.

Modafinil: Overall improvement in cognitive functioning was mixed across and within the three studies reviewed. All three studies reported modafinil improved cognitive performance on some tests, including psychomotor ability (Lundorff et al., 2009), information processing speed (Lundorff et al., 2009), and speed of memory and quality of episodic memory (Kohli et al., 2009). However, one study failed to find significant improvement in learning and memory, fine motor ability, and verbal fluency (Blackhall et al., 2009), and another study failed to document significant improvement in continuity of attention (Kohli et al., 2009). Based on these mixed results, further randomized controlled trials are warranted to determine efficacy.

COMPLEMENTARY AND ALTERNATIVE MEDICINE

Four studies using two categories of complementary and alternative medicine (CAM) interventions were found testing vitamin E (Chan, Cheung, Law, & Chan, 2004; Jatoi et al., 2005) or exercise (Korstjens, Mesters, van der Peet, Gijsen, & van den Borne, 2006; Schwartz et al., 2002). Within each CAM category, one of the studies combined the CAM intervention with a medication: vitamin E with donepezil (Jatoi et al., 2005) and exercise with methylphenidate (Schwartz et al., 2002). Results of these studies are equivocal, thus limiting the conclusions that can be made. Further replication and incorporation of randomized clinical trials are recommended.

Exercise

Two nonrandomized trials examined the impact of exercise on cognitive function as a secondary outcome (Korstjens et al., 2006; Schwartz et al., 2002). In a small prospective trial, Schwartz and colleagues (2002) combined an exercise program with administration of methylphenidate. After four months, improvements in physical performance as measured by a 12-minute walk were associated with greater improvements in visual attention, motor speed, and cognitive flexibility. In a larger trial, Korstjens and colleagues (2006) observed improvements in cognitive function after three months of exercise and an educational program on fatigue. Cognitive function was measured by two self-reported items with no objective measures used. Although exercise may be a promising intervention for cognitive function, replication with comparison groups and objective measures is warranted.

Vitamin E

Mixed results were observed in the two small studies examining the use of vitamin E for cognitive function (Chan et al., 2004; Jatoi et al., 2005). Using a quasi-experimental design, 1,000 IU of vitamin E was administered twice daily over a one-year duration (Chan et al., 2004). Improvements in global cognition, verbal and visual memory (including immediate and delayed recall), and executive function were observed for those receiving treatment. However, Jatoi and colleagues (2005) conducted a randomized, controlled, double-blind, placebo-controlled trial and failed to find a significant effect of 5 mg/day donepezil and 1,000 IU/day vitamin E on cognitive functioning after administration over three months. Differences in design and methods may contribute to these equivocal results; therefore, replication with a large randomized controlled trial is recommended.

COGNITIVE TRAINING PROGRAM INTERVENTIONS

Six studies have examined the use of cognitive training programs for improving cognitive function during or upon completion of cancer treatment (Ferguson et al., 2007; Gehring et al., 2009; Locke et al., 2008; McDougall, 2001; Poppelreuter, Weis, & Bartsch, 2009; Sherer, Meyers, & Bergloff, 1997). Cognitive training programs vary according to the design, personnel, involvement with caregivers, and duration, limiting conclusions across studies and warranting further study. Cognitive training programs involved computerized programs (Ferguson et al., 2007; Gehring et al., 2009; Poppelreuter et al., 2009) or sessions with trained personnel (Locke et al., 2008; McDougall, 2001; Sherer et al., 1997) and were most commonly aimed at memory, attention, or executive function. All programs offered concurrent psychoeducational training directed to incorporate compensatory skills into daily function. Although these cognitive training programs appear positive, five studies were limited by small sample size and lack of comparison groups (Ferguson et al., 2007; Locke et al., 2008; McDougall, 2001; Poppelreuter et al., 2009; Sherer et al., 1997).

Three studies used computerized programs in the delivery of cognitive training for a duration ranging from six weeks to four months (Ferguson et al., 2007; Gehring et al., 2009; Poppelreuter et al., 2009). Although some observed sustained improvements in verbal memory (Ferguson et al., 2007; Gehring et al., 2009), attention (Gehring et al., 2009), and executive control function (Ferguson et al., 2007), trends toward improving memory and attention were not maintained throughout program duration in one study (Poppelreuter et al., 2009).

Three studies used trained personnel to deliver individualized or group cognitive training and psychoeducational programs. Although McDougall (2001) did not observe any objectively measured sustained improvements in memory, subjects reported sustained improvements. Similarly, sustained use of compensatory skills gained from training (Locke et al., 2008) and improvements in independent functioning (Sherer et al., 1997) observed after training completion may reflect improvements in some cognitive domains; however, both studies failed to use objective measures for cognitive function.

Effectiveness Unlikely

Interventions for which lack of effectiveness has been demonstrated by negative evidence from a single rigorously conducted controlled trial, consistent negative evidence from well-designed controlled trials using small samples, or guidelines developed from evidence and supported by expert opinion

There are no interventions as of February 2010.

Not Recommended for Practice

Interventions for which lack of effectiveness or harmfulness has been demonstrated by strong evidence from rigorously conducted studies, meta-analyses, or systematic reviews, or interventions where the costs, burden, or harms associated with the intervention exceed anticipated benefit

EPOETIN ALFA

Seven studies (Chang, Couture, Young, Lau, & McWatters, 2004; Iconomou et al., 2008; Mancuso, Migliorino, De Santis, Saponiero, & DeMarinis, 2006; Mar Fan et al., 2009; Massa, Madeddu, Lusso, Gramignano, & Mantovani, 2006; O'Shaughnessy, 2002; O'Shaughnessy et al., 2005) were found that evaluated the use of erythropoiesis-stimulating agents (ESAs) to improve cognitive functioning in patients receiving chemotherapy. Although two studies (Chang et al., 2004; Massa et al., 2006) reported improvement in cognitive function, other studies failed to demonstrate any significant effects of ESAs on cognitive functioning. Although these studies had several methodologic limitations, further investigation would not be recommended because of U.S. Food and Drug Administration warnings regarding risks associated with the use of ESAs. These safety concerns include the risk of increased tumor growth, decreased survival, and increased cardiovascular side effects.

Expert Opinion

Low-risk interventions that are (1) consistent with sound clinical practice, (2) suggested by an expert in a peer-reviewed publication (journal or book chapter), and (3) for which limited evidence exists. An expert is an individual with peer-reviewed journal publications in the domain of interest.

There are no interventions as of February 2010.

Areas for Research

Cognitive impairment in patients with cancer may be disruptive, bothersome, and potentially debilitating (Mehnert et al., 2007; Von Ah, Russell, Storniolo, & Carpenter, 2009). Although research in this area has grown significantly in the last few years, especially for patients with brain tumors or breast cancer, more work is needed. Focused research regarding cognitive impairment in patients with cancer is needed in the following areas.
- Understanding the prevalence and trajectory of cognitive impairment across various types of patients with cancer and treatment regimens.
- Identifying potential predictors of cognitive impairment so that patients at risk may be identified and treated sooner. This would include identifying factors that may predispose individual patients with cancer for cognitive impairment, such as genetic polymorphisms.
- Developing assessment instruments that are reliable, valid, sensitive to subtle changes, and easily implemented in the clinical setting. This is critical for identifying and treating patients efficiently.
- Identifying the underlying physiologic mechanisms associated with cognitive impairment in patients with cancer so that effective preventive or treatment strategies may be developed.
- Developing and testing evidence-based and cost-effective treatment options that are amenable to patients with cancer.
- Identifying symptoms associated with cognitive impairment (e.g., pain, sleep disturbance, fatigue, depression) that if left untreated may exacerbate the problem and thwart effective treatment.

Overall, research in the area of cancer- and cancer treatment–related cognitive impairment has grown. However, large, well-designed, randomized controlled trials are needed to improve understanding of this symptom and to identify the best methods of treatment.

Search Strategy

Computerized literature searching was done using the consolidated PICO (Patient/Problem, Intervention, Comparison, and Outcome) terms that are outlined as follows. An initial date range of 10 years was used, and additional manual retrieval was done for key findings from the literature. The limitations of adults and English language were used. The final literature search for evidence related to interventions was performed in February 2010.

Patient/Problem: Patients with cancer who have cognitive impairment, cognitive deficits, or cognitive dysfunction, including memory changes or dysfunction, chemotherapy-related cognitive changes, changes in attention, concentration, executive function, visuospatial skills, language, motor skills, information processing and speed, and delirium in advanced cancer

Intervention: Stimulants, including d-methylphenidate (Ritalin®, Novartis Pharmaceuticals), modafinil (Provigil®, Cephalon), donepezil, and erythropoietin; memory and adaptation training; energy conservation and restorative activities; environmental interventions; meditation;

exercise; neuropsychiatric rehabilitation; herbals and vitamins; complementary and alternative interventions, including ginseng, ginkgo biloba, vitamin E, and acupuncture; and other medications, including statins, monoamine oxidase inhibitors, and angiotensin-converting enzyme inhibitors

Comparison: Standard care

Outcome: Improvement in cognitive function: memory, attention, concentration, executive function, visuospatial skills, motor skills, information processing and speed. Improvement in energy/fatigue, energy conservation. Improved ability to compensate for memory problems. Improvement in self-reported and cognitive test results. Improvement in quality of life.

Type of Question: Prevention or treatment

Databases Used: ProQuest Nursing Basic, PubMed, CINAHL®, EMBASE®, Cochrane Collaboration

Inclusion Criteria: Clinical intervention study, adults, patients with cancer

Definitions of the interventions are available at **www.ons.org/research/PEP**.
Literature search completed through February 2010.

References

Blackhall, L., Petroni, G., Shu, J., Baum, L., & Farace, E. (2009). A pilot study evaluating the safety and efficacy of modafinil for cancer-related fatigue. *Journal of Palliative Medicine, 12,* 433–439. doi:10.1089/jpm.2008.0230

Bruera, E., Miller, M.J., Macmillan, K., & Kuehn, N. (1992). Neuropsychological effects of methylphenidate in patients receiving a continuous infusion of narcotics for cancer pain. *Pain, 48,* 163–166.

Butler, J.M., Case, L.D., Atkins, J., Frizzell, B., Sanders, G., Griffin, P., … Shaw, E.G. (2007). A phase III, double-blind, placebo-controlled prospective randomized clinical trial of d-threo-methylphenidate HCl in brain tumor patients receiving radiation therapy. *International Journal of Radiation Oncology, Biology, Physics, 69,* 1496–1501. doi:10.1016/j.ijrobp.2007.05.076

Chan, A.S., Cheung, M.-C., Law, S.C., & Chan, J.H. (2004). Phase II study of alpha-tocopherol in improving the cognitive function of patients with temporal lobe radionecrosis. *Cancer, 100,* 398–401. doi:10.1002/cncr.11885

Chang, J., Couture, F.A., Young, S.D., Lau, C.Y., & McWatters, K.L. (2004). Weekly administration of epoetin alfa improves cognition and quality of life in patients with breast cancer receiving chemotherapy. *Supportive Cancer Therapy, 2,* 52–58. doi:10.3816/SCT.2004.n.023

Ferguson, R.J., Ahles, T.A., Saykin, A.J., McDonald, B.C., Furstenberg, C.T., Cole, B.F., & Mott, L.A. (2007). Cognitive-behavioral management of chemotherapy related cognitive change. *Psycho-Oncology, 16,* 772–777. doi:10.1002/pon.1133

Gagnon, B., Low, G., & Schreier, G. (2005). Methylphenidate hydrochloride improves cognitive function in patients with advanced cancer and hypoactive delirium: A prospective clinical study. *Journal of Psychiatry and Neuroscience, 30,* 100–107. Retrieved from http://www.ncbi.nlm.nih.gov/pmc/articles/PMC551162/?tool=pubmed

Gehring, K., Sitskoorn, M.M., Gundy, C.M., Sikkes, S.A.M., Klein, M., Postma, T.J., … Aaronson, N.K. (2009). Cognitive rehabilitation in patients with gliomas: A randomized, controlled trial. *Journal of Clinical Oncology, 27,* 3712–3722. doi:10.1200/JCO.2008.20.5765

Iconomou, G., Koutras, A., Karaivazoglou, K., Kalliolas, G.D., Assimakopoulos, K., Argyriou, A.A., … Kalofonos, H.P. (2008). Effect of epoetin alfa therapy on cognitive function in anaemic patients with solid tumours undergoing chemotherapy. *European Journal of Cancer Care, 17,* 535–541. doi:10.1111/j.1365.2354.2007.00857x

Jatoi, A., Kahanic, S.P., Frytak, S.P., Schaefer, P., Foote, R.L., Sloan, J., & Petersen, R.C. (2005). Donepezil and vitamin E for preventing cognitive dysfunction in small cell lung cancer patients: Preliminary results and suggestions for future study designs. *Supportive Care in Cancer, 13,* 66–69. doi:10.1007/s00520-004-0696-0

Kohli, S., Fisher, S.G., Tra, Y., Adams, J., Mapstone, M.E., Wesnes, K.A., … Morrow, G.R. (2009). The effects of modafinil on cognitive function in breast cancer survivors. *Cancer, 115,* 2605–2616. doi:10.1002/cncr.24287

Korstjens, I., Mesters, I., van der Peet, E., Gijsen, B., & van den Borne, B. (2006). Quality of life of cancer survivors after physical and psychosocial rehabilitation. *European Journal of Cancer Prevention, 15,* 541–547. doi:10.1097/01.cej.0000220625.77857.95

Locke, D., Cerhan, J., Wu, W., Malec, J., Clark, M.M., Rummans, T.A., & Brown, P.D. (2008). Cognitive rehabilitation and problem-solving to improve quality of life of patients with primary brain tumors: A pilot study. *Journal of Supportive Oncology, 6,* 383–391.

Lower, E.E., Fleishman, S., Cooper, A., Zeldis, J., Faleck, H., Yu, Z., & Manning, D. (2009). Efficacy of dexmethylphenidate for the treatment of fatigue after cancer chemotherapy: A randomized clinical trial. *Journal of Pain and Symptom Management, 38,* 650–662. doi:10.1016/j.jpainsymman.2009.03.011

Lundorff, L.E., Jønsson, B.H., & Sjøgren, P. (2009). Modafinil for attentional and psychomotor dysfunction in advanced cancer: A double-blind randomised, cross-over trial. *Palliative Medicine, 23,* 731–738. doi:10.1177/0269216309106872

Mancuso, A., Migliorino, M., De Santis, S., Saponiero, A., & DeMarinis, F. (2006). Correlation between anemia and functional/cognitive capacity in elderly lung cancer patients treated with chemotherapy. *Annals of Oncology 17,* 146–150. doi:10.1093/annonc/mdj038

Mar Fan, H.G., Clemons, M., Xu, W., Chemerynsky, I., Breunis, H., Braganza, S., & Tannock, I.F. (2008). A randomised, placebo-controlled, double-blind trial of the effects of d-methylphenidate on fatigue and cognitive dysfunction in women undergoing adjuvant chemotherapy for breast cancer. *Supportive Care in Cancer, 16,* 577–583. doi:10.1007/s00520-007-0341-9

Mar Fan, H.G., Park, A., Xu, W., Yi, Q.-L., Braganza, S., Chang, J., … Tannock, I.F. (2009). The influence of erythropoietin on cognitive function in women following chemotherapy for breast cancer. *Psycho-Oncology, 18,* 156–161. doi:10.1002/pon.1372

Massa, E., Madeddu, C., Lusso, M.R., Gramignano, G., & Mantovani, G. (2006). Evaluation of the effectiveness of treatment with erythropoietin on anemia, cognitive functioning and functions studied by comprehensive geriatric assessment in elderly cancer patients with anemia related to cancer chemotherapy. *Critical Reviews in Oncology/Hematology, 57,* 175–182. doi:10.1016/j.critrevonc.2005.06.001

McDougall, G.J., Jr. (2001). Memory improvement program for elderly cancer survivors. *Geriatric Nursing, 22,* 185–190. doi:10.1067/mgn.2001.117916

Mehnert, A., Scherwath, A., Schirmer, L., Schleimer, B., Petersen, C., Schulz-Kindermann, F., … Koch, U. (2007). The association between neuropsychological impairment, self-perceived cognitive deficits, fatigue and health related quality of life in breast cancer survivors following standard adjuvant versus high-dose chemotherapy. *Patient Education and Counseling, 66,* 108–118. doi:10.1016/j.pec.2006.11.005

Meyers, C.A., Weitzner, M.A., Valentine, A.D., & Levin, V.A. (1998). Methylphenidate therapy improves cognition, mood, and function of brain tumor patients. *Journal of Clinical Oncology, 16,* 2522–2527.

O'Shaughnessy, J.A. (2002). Effects of epoetin alfa on cognitive function, mood, asthenia, and quality of life in women with breast cancer undergoing adjuvant chemotherapy. *Clinical Breast Cancer, 3*(Suppl. 3), S116–S120.

O'Shaughnessy, J.A., Vukelja, S.J., Holmes, F.A., Savin, M., Jones, M., Royall, D., … Von Hoff, D. (2005). Feasibility of quantifying the effects of epoetin alfa therapy on cognitive function in women with breast cancer undergoing adjuvant or neoadjuvant chemotherapy. *Clinical Breast Cancer, 5,* 439–446.

Poppelreuter, M., Weis, J., & Bartsch, H.H. (2009). Effects of specific neuropsychological training programs for breast cancer patients after adjuvant chemotherapy. *Journal of Psychosocial Oncology, 27,* 274–296. doi:10.1080/07347330902776044

Schwartz, A.L., Thompson, J.A., & Masood, N. (2002). Interferon-induced fatigue in patients with melanoma: A pilot study of exercise and methylphenidate [Online exclusive]. *Oncology Nursing Forum, 29,* E85–E90. doi:10.1188/02.ONF.E85-E90

Shaw, E.G., Rosdhal, R., D'Agostino, R.B., Lovato, J., Naughton, M.J., Robbins, M.E., & Rapp, S.R. (2006). Phase II study of donepezil in irradiated brain tumor patients: Effect on cognitive function, mood, and quality of life. *Journal of Clinical Oncology, 24,* 1415–1420. doi:10.1200/JCO.2005.03.3001

Sherer, M., Meyers, C.A., & Bergloff, P. (1997). Efficacy of postacute brain injury rehabilitation for patients with primary malignant brain tumors. *Cancer, 80,* 250–257. doi:10.1002/(SICI)1097-0142(19970715)80:2<250::AID-CNCR13>3.0.CO;2-T

Von Ah, D., Russell, K., Storniolo, A.M., & Carpenter, J.S. (2009). Cognitive dysfunction and its relationship to quality of life in breast cancer survivors. *Oncology Nursing Forum, 36,* 326–334. doi:10.1188/09.ONF.326-334

CHAPTER 3

Hot Flashes

Editor, Marcelle Kaplan, RN, MS, AOCN®, CBCN®

Problem

A *hot flash* is defined as "a subjective sensation of heat that is associated with objective signs of cutaneous vasodilation and a subsequent drop in core temperature" (Boekhout, Beijnen, & Schellens, 2006, p. 642). Synonyms for this experience include *hot flushes, vasomotor symptoms, night sweats,* and *menopausal symptoms.* Hot flashes may be accompanied by facial flushing, perspiration, chills, heart palpitations, night sweats, and feelings of anxiety (Boekhout et al., 2006; Finck, Barton, Loprinzi, Quella, & Sloan, 1998). The frequency, duration, and intensity of hot flashes can vary widely. They have been reported to occur as infrequently as several times a month to as often as every hour and may last for a few seconds to several minutes. Hot flash intensity can be characterized as mild, moderate, severe, or very severe (Finck et al., 1998).

Hot flashes are significantly more frequent and severe in women diagnosed with breast cancer than in women without the disease and are common in breast cancer survivors following adjuvant treatment (Carpenter, 2000). In the adjuvant treatment setting, studies have shown that agents used to suppress ovarian function and cause estrogen withdrawal, such as tamoxifen and aromatase inhibitors, increase the frequency and severity of hot flashes and that hot flashes are reported as the most common adverse effect associated with these agents (Howell et al., 2005).

Men being treated for prostate cancer with androgen deprivation, hormonal therapies, or surgical castration also commonly experience vasomotor symptoms with hot flashes and sweating (Lee, Kim, Shin, Choi, & Ernst, 2009).

For the purposes of this chapter, the literature search was confined to evidence-based interventions for managing hot flashes in women with breast cancer and men with prostate cancer.

Pathophysiology of Hot Flashes

The etiology of hot flashes is unknown. One hypothesis is that decreases in estrogen levels in women or gonadal hormone levels in men lead to increases in the plasma levels of the neurotransmitters norepinephrine and serotonin, which are thought to have important roles in thermoregulation. The effect of the changes in the plasma levels of these neurotransmitters is a lowering of the central thermoregulatory set point located in the hypothalamus, resulting in vasodilation and the hot flash sensation (Boekhout et al., 2006; Stearns, 2004).

Incidence

In healthy women, hot flashes rarely occur before women enter the perimenopausal transition and occur in a higher percentage of women in the later phases of the menopausal transition. Hot flashes occur with a higher frequency and greater severity in younger women who undergo a sudden onset of menopause due to surgical removal of their ovaries or medical conditions or treatments that decrease the ovaries' ability to produce hormones. In healthy women, the estimates of the prevalence of vasomotor symptoms vary from 14% to 51% in premenopausal women, from 35% to 50% in perimenopausal women, and from 30% to 80% in postmenopausal women (National Institutes of Health, 2005).

Cancer treatment, especially for breast cancer, can lead to both an earlier onset of menopause and exacerbation of existing menopausal symptoms. Hot flashes occur in more than 78% of all breast cancer survivors (Fenlon, Corner, & Haviland, 2008; Jacobson et al., 2001; Savard, Savard, Quesnel, & Ivers, 2009). At least 40% and as many as 59% of women with a cancer diagnosis rate their hot flashes as moderate or severe (Stearns, 2004; Tremblay, Sheeran, & Aranda, 2008).

In premenopausal women with breast cancer, adjuvant chemotherapy can cause premature ovarian failure and temporary or permanent amenorrhea. The incidence of chemotherapy-induced ovarian failure depends on the regimen used, cumulative drug doses, and the patient's age. Chemotherapy-induced ovarian failure causes symptoms similar to natural menopause and is associated with decreased circulating levels of estrogen and progesterone and increased levels of follicle-stimulating hormone and luteinizing hormone. Women with chemotherapy-induced menopause experience rapid changes in hormone concentrations and more severe symptoms than those associated with the more gradual decline in estrogen concentrations during normal aging (Baber, Hickey, & Kwik, 2005). The combination of chemotherapy and endocrine therapy causes premature menopause in more than 80% of premenopausal women during the first year after their diagnosis. More than 90% of women undergoing a bilateral oophorectomy will experience hot flashes that are severe and long lasting (Baber et al., 2005). As many as 78% of female chemotherapy recipients and 72% of tamoxifen recipients experience hot flashes (Elkins et al., 2008). Hot flashes are also among the most commonly reported symptoms in women receiving systemic therapy for breast cancer, adversely affecting quality of life (Pandya et al., 2005).

Approximately one-third of the healthy aging male population experience hot flashes, and 50% of these men find the symptoms to be bothersome (Adelson, Loprinzi, & Hershman, 2005). Hot flashes and sweating are common symptoms in men with advanced prostate cancer who have been surgically castrated (bilateral orchiectomy) or medically castrated by the use of gonadotropin-releasing hormone analogs. Hot flashes have been reported in 35%–80% of men who have been treated with androgen deprivation therapy (ADT) for advanced prostate cancer (Frisk, 2010).

Survivorship and Late Effects

Very few of the studies reviewed included any long-term follow-up. Randomized clinical trials with long-term follow-up are needed in both men and women to determine the long-term negative effects of these interventions. Hot flashes are often associated with sleep disturbance and diminished cognitive function, which can negatively affect quality of life (Engstrom, 2008). Spetz, Zetterlund, Varenhorst, and Hammar (2003) have reported that hot flashes may persist in at least 40% of men who have been treated with ADT for advanced prostate cancer for at least eight years after treatment. The eight-year duration of hot flashes has been demonstrated in several other studies as well (Frisk, 2010). The persistence of their distress has led men to discontinue ADT.

Hot flashes are more common in breast cancer survivors than in the general female population for a few reasons. Treatment with chemotherapy and hormonal therapies, such as tamoxifen or aromatase inhibitors, is associated with an increased incidence of hot flashes. In younger women treated with a combination of chemotherapy and endocrine therapy, as many as 80% will experience premature menopause in the first year after diagnosis (Baber et al., 2005). In addition, estrogen replacement therapy, which can alleviate hot flashes, is contraindicated in breast cancer survivors because of fears of stimulating disease recurrence (Loprinzi et al., 2000).

Because of the increasing number of breast cancer survivors, quality-of-life issues in this population have become increasingly significant. Women who experience hot flashes secondary to tamoxifen or other hormonal treatments may decide to discontinue treatment prematurely because of these side effects, thus losing the potential survival benefit. Five years of tamoxifen use is associated with a 50% reduction in risk of breast cancer recurrence (Batur, Blixen, Moore, Thacker, & Xu, 2006); however, early discontinuation rates of tamoxifen have been reported to range from 15% to 35%, especially in women reporting side effects (Buijs et al., 2009). Thus, developing strategies to control the vasomotor side effects of hormonal therapies is crucial to increase treatment compliance and potentially improve survival.

At the same time, it is also necessary to be cognizant of drug interactions that may decrease the efficacy of breast cancer therapies. Pharmacogenomic studies have identified a potential reduction in the effectiveness of tamoxifen when used with drugs that inhibit its bioactivation by the enzyme system cytochrome P450 2D6 (CYP2D6) (Henry, Stearns, Flockhart, Hayes, & Riba, 2008). Selective serotonin reuptake inhibitors (SSRIs), including venlafaxine, fluoxetine, and paroxetine, are antidepressant drugs that show promise in alleviating hot flashes. However, a number of studies that have specifically looked at SSRIs and the degree to which they inhibit CYP2D6 have demonstrated that fluoxetine and paroxetine are strong CYP2D6 inhibitors and should be avoided by women taking tamoxifen. Retrospective review of data indicates a potential for increased rates of breast cancer recurrence and decreased relapse-free survival for women taking tamoxifen with concurrent use of these strong inhibitors (Henry et al., 2008; Kelly et al., 2010).

Assessment and Clinical Measurement Tools

Hot flashes, a subjective experience, have been predominately measured in clinical trials through the use of patient self-reported diaries. No standard hot flash diary exists, but most diary logs include recording of hot flash frequency and severity. In an effort to objectively measure hot flashes, electronic monitoring devices that assess skin temperatures have been used as a hot flash measurement instrument (Carpenter, 2005). However, controversy exists regarding both objective and subjective hot flash measurement approaches (see Table 3-1).

The Placebo Effect on Hot Flashes

In interpreting data results from hot flash intervention studies, awareness of the placebo effect on reported symptoms is prudent. Subjects in numerous studies receiving placebo intervention have reported significant reductions in hot flash activity (Boekhout et al., 2006). About 25% of these participants reported at least a 50% reduction in hot flash episodes, and 15% reported a more than 75% hot flash reduction (Sloan et al., 2001).

In a review of the data from 375 subjects in seven randomized clinical trials that had a placebo arm, investigators found that those receiving the placebo intervention reported an average decrease in both hot flash frequency and hot flash scores of 25% at four weeks. The beneficial placebo effect was found to be consistent among another five randomized clinical trials of the North Central Cancer Treatment Group as well (Sloan et al., 2001). Thus, the placebo effect should be considered in relation to anecdotal reports regarding new interventions for hot flashes.

Table 3-1. Objective and Subjective Hot Flash Measurement Tools

Name of Tool	Number of Items	Domains	Reliability and Validity	Populations	Clinical Utility
Sternal skin conductance	Not applicable	Frequency	Validity established in laboratory setting	Men with prostate cancer; women with breast cancer	Unable to differentiate between hot flashes and other factors causing sweating in clinical setting
Hot flash diaries	Varied	Frequency and severity	Reliability and validity not established	Aging menopausal women; menopausal women with breast cancer	Convenient and inexpensive; subject to recall bias

References

Adelson, K.B., Loprinzi, C.L., & Hershman, D.L. (2005). Treatment of hot flushes in breast and prostate cancer. *Expert Opinion on Pharmacotherapy, 6,* 1095–1106. doi:10.1517/14656566.6.7.1095

Baber, R., Hickey, M., & Kwik, M. (2005). Therapy for menopausal symptoms during and after treatment for breast cancer: Safety considerations. *Drug Safety, 28,* 1085–1100.

Batur, P., Blixen, C., Moore, H., Thacker, H., & Xu, M. (2006). Menopausal hormone therapy (HT) in patients with breast cancer. *Maturitas, 53,* 123–132. doi:10.1016/j.maturitas.2005.03.004

Boekhout, A.H., Beijnen, J.H., & Schellens, J.H.M. (2006). Symptoms and treatment in cancer therapy-induced early menopause. *Oncologist, 11,* 641–654. doi:10.1634/theoncologist.11-6-641

Buijs, C., Mom, C.H., Willemse, P.H., Boezen, H.M., Maurer, J.M., Wymenga, A.N., … Mourits, M.J. (2009). Venlafaxine versus clonidine for the treatment of hot flashes in breast cancer patients: A double-blind, randomized cross-over study. *Breast Cancer Research and Treatment, 115,* 573–580. doi:10.1007/s10549-008-0138-7

Carpenter, J.S. (2000). Hot flashes and their management in breast cancer. *Seminars in Oncology Nursing, 16,* 214–225.

Carpenter, J.S. (2005). State of the science: Hot flashes and cancer, part 1: Definition, scope, impact, physiology, and measurement. *Oncology Nursing Forum, 32,* 959–968. doi:10.1188/04.ONF.959-968

Elkins, G., Marcus, J., Stearns, V., Perfect, M., Rajab, M.H., Ruud, C., … Keith, T. (2008). Randomized trial of a hypnosis intervention for treatment of hot flashes among breast cancer survivors. *Journal of Clinical Oncology, 26,* 5022–5026. doi:10.1200/JCO.2008.16.6389

Engstrom, C.A. (2008). Hot flashes in prostate cancer: State of the science. *American Journal of Men's Health, 2,* 122–132. doi:10.1177/1557988306298802

Fenlon, D.R., Corner, J.L., & Haviland, J.S. (2008). A randomized controlled trial of relaxation training to reduce hot flashes in women with primary breast cancer. *Journal of Pain and Symptom Management, 35,* 397–405. doi:10.1016/j.jpainsymman.2007.05.014

Finck, G., Barton, D.L., Loprinzi, C.L., Quella, S.K., & Sloan, J.A. (1998). Definitions of hot flashes in breast cancer survivors. *Journal of Pain and Symptom Management, 16,* 327–333. doi:10.1016/S0885-3924(98)00090-6

Frisk, J. (2010). Managing hot flushes in men after prostate cancer—A systematic review. *Maturitas, 65,* 15–22. doi:10.1016/j.maturitas.2009.10.017

Henry, N.L., Stearns, V., Flockhart, D.A., Hayes, D.F., & Riba, M. (2008). Drug interactions and pharmacogenomics in the treatment of breast cancer and depression. *American Journal of Psychiatry, 165,* 1251–1255. doi:10.1176/appi.ajp.2008.08040482

Howell, A., Cuzick, J., Baum, M., Buzdar, A., Dowsett, M., Forbes, J.F., … ATAC Trialists' Group. (2005). Results of the ATAC (arimidex, tamoxifen, alone or in combination) trial after completion of 5 years' adjuvant treatment for breast cancer. *Lancet, 365,* 60–62. doi:10.1016/S0140-6736(04)17666-6

Jacobson, J.S., Troxel, A.B., Evans, J., Klaus, L., Vahdat, L., Kinne, D., … Grann, V.R. (2001). Randomized trial of black cohosh for the treatment of hot flashes among women with a history of breast cancer. *Journal of Clinical Oncology, 19,* 2739–2745. Retrieved from http://jco.ascopubs.org/cgi/reprint/19/10/2739

Kelly, C., Juurlink, D., Gomes, T., Duong-Hua, M., Pritchard, K., Austin, P., & Paszat, L. (2010). Selective serotonin reuptake inhibitors and breast cancer mortality in women. *BMJ, 340,* c693. doi:10.1136/bmj.c693

Lee, S.L., Kim, K.-H., Shin, B.-C., Choi, S.-M., & Ernst, E. (2009). Acupuncture for treating hot flushes in men with prostate cancer: A systematic review. *Supportive Care in Cancer, 17,* 763–770. doi:10.1007/s00520-009-0589-3

Loprinzi, C.L., Kugler, J.W., Sloan, J.A., Mailliard, J.A., LaVasseur, B.I., Barton, D.L., … Christensen, B.J. (2000). Venlafaxine in management of hot flashes in survivors of breast cancer: A randomised controlled trial. *Lancet, 356,* 2059–2063. doi:10.1016/S0140-6736(00)03403-6

National Institutes of Health. (2005). NIH state-of-the-science conference statement on management of menopause-related symptoms. *NIH Consensus and State-of-the-Science Statements, 22,* 1–38.

Pandya, K.J., Morrow, G.R., Roscoe, J.A., Zhao, H., Hickok, J.T., Pajon, E., … Flynn, P.J. (2005). Gabapentin for hot flashes in 420 women with breast cancer: A randomised double-blind placebo-controlled trial. *Lancet, 366,* 818–824. doi:10.1016/S0140-6736(05)67215-7

Savard, M.H., Savard, J., Quesnel, C., & Ivers, H. (2009). The influence of breast cancer treatment on the occurrence of hot flashes. *Journal of Pain and Symptom Management, 37,* 687–697. doi:10.1016/j.jpainsymman.2008.04.010

Sloan, J.A., Loprinzi, C.L., Novotny, P.J., Barton, D.L., Lavasseur, B.I., & Windschitl, H. (2001). Methodologic lessons learned from hot flash studies. *Journal of Clinical Oncology, 19,* 4280–4290. Retrieved from http://jco.ascopubs.org/cgi/reprint/19/23/4280

Spetz, A.C., Zetterlund, E.L., Varenhorst, E., & Hammar, M. (2003). Incidence and management of hot flashes in prostate cancer. *Journal of Supportive Oncology, 1,* 263–273.

Stearns, V. (2004). Management of hot flashes in breast cancer survivors and men with prostate cancer. *Current Oncology Reports, 6,* 285–290.

Tremblay, A., Sheeran, L., & Aranda, S.K. (2008). Psychoeducational interventions to alleviate hot flashes: A systematic review. *Menopause, 15,* 193–202. doi:10.1097/gme.0b013e31805c08dc

Case Study

K.V. is a 38-year-old woman who was diagnosed with stage II breast carcinoma (T1cN1aM0 [grade 2, 1.6 cm tumor, 1 of 10 positive lymph nodes, estrogen receptor/progesterone receptor positive, HER2/neu negative]). K.V.'s oncologist recommended TAC (six cycles of doxorubicin, cyclophosphamide, and docetaxel every three weeks). K.V. is married and has three sons ranging in age from three to nine years old. K.V. also works part time as a certified public accountant. She had no prior history of breast biopsies and no family history of breast or ovarian cancer. She had been on oral contraceptives but has had no other estrogen exposure.

K.V. met with the oncology nurse prior to starting her treatment to discuss chemotherapy and side effects. She was very concerned about caring for her sons and keeping up with her family responsibilities and role as a mother and wife. In addition, she loved her job and wanted to keep working. During the teaching session, K.V. asked if her menses would stop during chemotherapy. The nurse told her that most likely chemotherapy would give her amenorrhea; however, being young, her menses would probably resume once chemotherapy was completed. K.V. was elated and stated, "No period! Great! This is so much to handle, and that is one thing I can live without!"

K.V. started her chemotherapy the following week. She did very well with minimal side effects. She was fatigued but still able to work part time and was grateful that her mother came to stay to help with the care of her sons.

Two days after her second cycle of chemotherapy, K.V. started menses. She was bleeding very heavily and became frightened that something was wrong, as her periods had never been this way in the past. K.V. called into the clinic to talk with the nurse. The nurse explained that her menses may be erratic with chemotherapy. K.V. was very upset and stated, "I was told I would have no periods during chemotherapy!" The nurse explained that this may happen but could take place after several chemotherapy cycles. The nurse instructed K.V. to call if her bleeding did not decrease in the next 24 hours. K.V.'s menses did stop within the next 24 hours, and she continued to do well.

After four cycles of chemotherapy, K.V. had no further menses. She was tired but determined to continue forward with treatment because as she stated, "I want to be here for my sons. This is not easy, but I will do it."

A few days before her fifth cycle, K.V. called into the clinic. She reported that she had a "horrible night." She told the nurse that she woke up drenched in sweat, was cold and clammy, and had heart palpitations. She got up to change her nightgown and found that she had no fever. She told the nurse that she had a similar episode that morning and wanted to know what was happening to her.

K.V. came to the clinic for blood work and to be evaluated. Her complete blood count was normal. After further discussion, K.V.'s diagnosis was hot flashes secondary to a chemotherapy-induced decrease in estrogen levels. K.V. was extremely depressed and crying. She stated, "I wanted my periods to stop, but I can't take these hot flashes. It is not fair; I am too young for hot flashes! Make them stop!"

The nurse immediately went to the ONS PEP resource on hot flashes to review interventions that would likely be effective. The nurse brought the list of pharmacologic agents to review with K.V. She stated that she did not want another pill and that her friend told her to take black cohosh because this had worked for her. The nurse reviewed the evidence from black cohosh and told K.V. that research suggests that this may not be as effective as pharmacologic agents. K.V. refused and stated that she was going to start taking black cohosh.

Two weeks later, K.V. again called the nurse. She stated that she was having hot flashes every two hours and was "miserable." She reported that the black cohosh did not work, and she was ready to take a pill. The nurse discussed this with the doctor, and he ordered paroxetine 20 mg per day. K.V. started her medication that day. When she returned for her sixth and final cycle of chemotherapy, her hot flashes were almost resolved. K.V. was very happy to be completing chemotherapy and to be rid of her hot flashes.

K.V. returned three weeks after completing chemotherapy to see the doctor and to discuss hormonal therapy because she was estrogen/progesterone receptor positive. Because she was only 38 years old, hormonal blood tests were performed, and they showed that K.V. was premenopausal. Although she was not currently having menses, these would probably return because she was finished with chemotherapy. The doctor prescribed tamoxifen but was concerned with the recent literature regarding the use of concomitant paroxetine and tamoxifen because of reports of increased risk of death related to breast cancer. The doctor told K.V. that he wanted her to stop the paroxetine. K.V. was very upset because she had no further hot flashes. The doctor agreed to start K.V. on venlafaxine, which was shown to be more effective for hot flashes. K.V. started tamoxifen and venlafaxine. At her four-week follow-up visit, K.V. had not experienced any hot flashes since changing medications and was tolerating tamoxifen. She was feeling less fatigued since completing chemotherapy and was happy that her hair was growing back.

Hot Flashes

AUTHORS
Marcelle Kaplan, RN, MS, AOCN®, CBCN®, Suzanne Mahon, RN, DNSc, AOCN®, APNG,
Diane Cope, RN, PhD, ARNP-BC, AOCNP®, Stacey Hill, RN, BSN,
Elizabeth Keating, RN, MS, NP, CBCN®, and Marcie Jacobson, RN, BSN, OCN®
LIBRARIANS: Andy Hickner, MSI, and Mark Vrabel, MLS, AHIP, ELS
ONS STAFF: Kristen Fessele, RN, MSN, ANP-BC, AOCN®

What interventions are effective in preventing and treating hot flashes in people with cancer?

Recommended for Practice

Interventions for which effectiveness has been demonstrated by strong evidence from rigorously conducted studies, meta-analyses, or systematic reviews and for which expectation of harms is small compared with the benefits

No interventions are recommended as of February 2010.

Likely to Be Effective

Interventions for which effectiveness has been demonstrated from a single rigorously conducted controlled trial, consistent supportive evidence from well-designed controlled trials using small samples, or guidelines developed from evidence and supported by expert opinion

PHARMACOLOGIC INTERVENTIONS

Gabapentin
Two randomized controlled trials of gabapentin versus placebo for treatment of hot flashes in women with breast cancer showed a significant difference in hot flashes with gabapentin 900 mg per day versus placebo (Loprinzi et al., 2009; Pandya et al., 2005).

One randomized controlled trial of gabapentin versus vitamin E for treatment of hot flashes in women with breast cancer showed a significant difference in hot flashes with gabapentin 900 mg/day versus vitamin E 800 IU/day (Biglia et al., 2007).

Venlafaxine
One double-blind, placebo-controlled, randomized trial showed that venlafaxine (Effexor®, Pfizer) can effectively reduce hot flashes and that the most appropriate dose for this indication is 75 mg per day. This trial included breast cancer survivors on tamoxifen (69%) and some healthy women (Loprinzi et al., 2000).

Two randomized crossover studies compared venlafaxine to clonidine and found both to be effective in relieving hot flashes (Buijs et al., 2009; Loibl et al., 2007).

One randomized double-blind, placebo-controlled crossover trial compared low-dose (37.5 mg) and high-dose (75 mg) venlafaxine and found that at both doses, venlafaxine resulted in modest hot flash reduction, and only hot flash interference improved differentially at the higher dose (Carpenter et al., 2007).

One open-label study reported that venlafaxine was effective at a low dose (37.5 mg) in relieving hot flashes. This small study was not blinded or placebo controlled (Biglia et al., 2005).

Benefits Balanced With Harms

Interventions for which clinicians and patients should weigh the beneficial and harmful effects according to individual circumstances and priorities

There are no interventions as of February 2010.

Effectiveness Not Established

Interventions for which insufficient or conflicting data or data of inadequate quality currently exist, with no clear indication of harm

PHARMACOLOGIC INTERVENTIONS

Clonidine
A randomized, double-blind, placebo-controlled trial evaluated oral clonidine 0.1 mg daily versus placebo for eight weeks in postmenopausal women receiving tamoxifen for breast cancer. Mean decrease in hot flash frequency was greater in the clonidine group than in the placebo group at four weeks (37% to 20%, respectively) and eight weeks (38% to 24%). Significant placebo effect was noted. Long-term effectiveness was not evaluated. No adverse effect on blood pressure was reported (Pandya et al., 2000).

One randomized, double-blind, crossover, prospective study compared transdermal clonidine to placebo for eight weeks in women experiencing tamoxifen-induced hot flashes. A clinically moderate decrease in hot flashes was reported from baseline in frequency (20%) and severity (10%) (Goldberg et al., 1994).

A small randomized, double-blind, crossover, prospective trial evaluating transdermal clonidine versus placebo for alleviating hot flashes in men with prostate cancer after orchiectomy found no significant benefit with clonidine (Loprinzi et al., 1994).

Estrogen Replacement Therapy (Men)
One small open-label crossover trial in men receiving leuprolide for prostate cancer evaluated two doses of transdermal estrogen. A significant reduction in the severity of hot flashes occurred with both doses. Serum testosterone levels showed no significant change (Gerber, Zagaja, Ray, & Rukstalis, 2000).

Fluoxetine
One phase III evaluation of fluoxetine (Prozac®, Eli Lilly) for treatment of hot flashes in women with a history of or an increased risk for breast cancer randomized subjects between fluoxetine (20 mg daily) and a placebo. This trial had fewer than 100 participants, and the results were not adjusted for potential confounding influences such as age or tamoxifen use. After five weeks of treatment, quality of life and occurrence of hot flashes did not differ between groups (Loprinzi et al., 2002).

Mirtazapine
One small pilot study evaluated the efficacy and safety of mirtazapine (Remeron®, Organon USA) 30 mg daily for 12 weeks to reduce hot flashes in women with breast cancer. Compared to baseline values, vasomotor symptoms decreased significantly (Biglia et al., 2007).

Paroxetine
One randomized controlled trial of paroxetine versus placebo for treatment of hot flashes in women with breast cancer showed a significant difference in hot flashes with paroxetine 10 mg per day and paroxetine 20 mg per day versus placebo (Stearns et al., 2005).

One retrospective study of women with breast cancer receiving tamoxifen therapy and concomitant use of a single selective serotonin reuptake inhibitor antidepressant showed significant increased risk of death from breast cancer with overlapping use of tamoxifen and paroxetine (Kelly et al., 2010).

Progestin Therapy
One phase III (Southwest Oncology Group study 9626) randomized, placebo-controlled, double-blind trial evaluated two doses of megestrol for women experiencing menopausal symptoms following a breast cancer diagnosis. At three months, the women showed a 65% improvement in symptoms with 20 mg daily, a 48% improvement in symptoms with 40 mg daily, and a significant placebo effect (14%). Duration of the effect continued at six months. Megestrol 20 mg daily is the recommended daily dose. Concern remains regarding the use of progestin in women with a history of breast cancer (Goodwin et al., 2008).

One double-blind, randomized crossover trial evaluated the use of megestrol 40 mg daily versus placebo for hot flash management in women with breast cancer or in men with prostate cancer who had undergone surgical or medical orchiectomy. At four weeks, an intention-to-treat analysis revealed a 74% reduction in hot flashes for patients receiving megestrol and a 21% reduction in the placebo group. No significant toxicities were reported (Loprinzi et al., 1994).

A small randomized trial compared intramuscular depot medroxyprogesterone (MPA) to oral megestrol for the control of hot flashes in women with breast cancer. Of the patients who received MPA, 75% responded to treatment, and 67% of those who received megestrol experienced a response. However, this was not considered to be statistically significant. The trial did not include a placebo group (Bertelli et al., 2002).

Sertraline
One double-blind, placebo-controlled crossover study evaluated sertraline (Zoloft®, Pfizer) versus placebo for treatment of hot flashes in women with early-stage breast cancer taking tamoxifen. Study subjects were given sertraline 50 mg every morning for six weeks followed by six weeks of placebo and then another six weeks of sertraline 50 mg. No statistically significant difference was found (Kimmick, Lovato, McQuellon, Robinson, & Muss, 2006).

Stellate Ganglion Block
A stellate ganglion block is an injection of local anesthetic in the sympathetic nerve tissue. Lipov et al. (2008) investigated the effectiveness of stellate ganglion block for the treatment of hot flashes in a small number of women with breast cancer (N = 13). At 12 weeks, hot flashes had decreased from a mean of 79 episodes per week prior to intervention to a mean of 8 episodes per week.

Testosterone Replacement Therapy

A retrospective review was conducted of 10 patients treated for prostate cancer who subsequently received testosterone replacement therapy (TRT) for symptoms of hypogonadism, including hot flashes. Median duration of therapy was 19 months, during which the number of hot flash episodes decreased and no recurrence of disease developed. However, a few case reports suggest that short-term TRT can cause an increase in prostate-specific antigen levels and convert an occult lesion into one that is clinically apparent (Agarwal & Oefelein, 2005).

Tibolone

One randomized, double-blind, placebo-controlled trial evaluated tibolone versus placebo in postmenopausal women receiving tamoxifen after surgery for breast cancer. Subjects were randomized to receive 20 mg per day of tamoxifen plus 2.5 mg per day of tibolone or placebo. Daily diaries showed no change in daily number of hot flashes with either tibolone or placebo after three months. The effect of tibolone on breast cancer recurrence is unknown (Kroiss et al., 2005).

COMPLEMENTARY AND SUPPLEMENT INTERVENTIONS

Acupuncture

Acupuncture is the procedure of inserting and manipulating needles into various points on the body to relieve pain or for other therapeutic purposes. It is typically administered by a trained acupuncturist but with training can be self-administered by some.

Six randomized trials of acupuncture in various groups demonstrated a decrease in hot flash occurrence (Deng et al., 2007; Filshie, Bolton, Browne, & Ashley, 2005; Frisk, Carlhall, Kallstrom, Lindh-Astrand, Malmstrom, & Hammar, 2008; Hervik & Mjåland, 2009; Nedstrand, Wijma, Wyon, & Hammar, 2005; Walker et al., 2010). Sample size was less than 72 total subjects in all studies. Follow-up was limited and in no study was for more than six months.

One pilot study of seven men who received acupuncture showed a decrease in hot flashes (follow-up was 10 weeks) (Hammar et al., 1999).

A convenience sample of 60 consecutive women receiving acupuncture for 10 weeks showed a decrease in hot flashes (Harding, Harris, & Chadwick, 2008).

A convenience sample of 12 women with breast cancer receiving tamoxifen showed some decrease in hot flashes (Towlerton, O'Brien, & Duncan, 1999).

Black Cohosh

Black cohosh is a perennial herb that grows in eastern North America. A substance obtained from the plant root has been used in some cultures to treat a variety of medical problems. It is being studied in the treatment of hot flashes and other symptoms of menopause (National Cancer Institute, n.d.).

Two double-blind controlled trials of black cohosh versus placebo did not show evidence that black cohosh reduced hot flashes more than the placebo (Jacobson et al., 2001; Pockaj et al., 2006). In the study stratified for tamoxifen use, differences in hot flash activity between the treatment and placebo groups, adjusted for tamoxifen, were not statistically significant (Jacobson et al., 2001). One randomized open-label study assessing the effect of black cohosh on tamoxifen-associated hot flash activity in young premenopausal breast cancer survivors showed that the combination of tamoxifen plus a black cohosh preparation significantly reduced the vasomotor episodes induced by tamoxifen in usual doses in breast cancer survivors over a 12-month period (Muñoz & Pluchino, 2003).

Hypnosis

Hypnosis is a form of relaxation therapy in which the person reaches a state of restful alertness with deeply focused concentration. The person can be relatively unaware of, but not completely blind to, his or her surroundings, and he or she may be more open to suggestion. It is provided by a trained hypnotherapist.

One randomly assigned trial of 60 women with breast cancer showed a decrease in hot flashes following hypnosis (Elkins et al., 2008). Follow-up was five weeks.

Three pilot studies, all with a sample size of 16 or fewer, showed a decrease in hot flashes (Elkins, Marcus, Palamara, & Stearns, 2004; Elkins, Marcus, Stearns, & Rajab, 2007; Younus, Simpson, Collins, & Wang, 2003).

Peer Counseling

Peer counseling can be provided by individuals who have experienced a certain situation or diagnosis and have received training on how to facilitate a group.

One randomized study of 60 African American women with breast cancer demonstrated a decrease in menopausal symptoms (Schover et al., 2006).

Relaxation Therapy

Relaxation therapy is a set of techniques to calm the body and mind. One trial of 150 women with breast cancer demonstrated a decrease in hot flashes (Fenlon, Corner, & Haviland, 2008). Attrition was significant (final sample size was 104), and follow-up was three months.

Vitamin E

One randomized, double-blind, crossover trial of vitamin E versus placebo, stratified by age and tamoxifen use, showed that vitamin E was associated with a minimal decrease in hot flashes (one less hot flash per day than was seen with a placebo) ($p \leq 0.05$). At the study end, subjects did not prefer vitamin E over the placebo, and no toxicity was demonstrated (Barton et al., 1998).

One randomized study assessed the efficacy and tolerability of gabapentin 900 mg/day for the control of vasomotor symptoms in women with breast cancer in comparison with vitamin E, which was used as a placebo-equivalent. This study was not blinded and did not include a placebo control arm. Results demonstrated that vitamin E had only a marginal effect on vasomotor symptoms; hot flash frequency and severity scores were reduced by 10.02% and 7.28%, respectively ($p \geq 0.05$). Gabapentin 900 mg/day was effective for relieving hot flashes in subjects previously treated for breast cancer (Biglia et al., 2009) (see Gabapentin).

Yoga

Yoga is a form of anaerobic exercise that involves a program of precise posture, breathing exercises, and meditation.

A randomized trial of 37 women who either received instruction in yoga techniques or were in a control group showed a decrease in hot flashes among women who received the instruction (Carson, Carson, Porter, Keefe, & Seewaldt, 2009). Follow-up was three months.

Effectiveness Unlikely

Interventions for which lack of effectiveness has been demonstrated by negative evidence from a single rigorously conducted controlled trial, consistent negative evidence from well-designed controlled trials using small samples, or guidelines developed from evidence and supported by expert opinion

HOMEOPATHY

The homeopathy approach to treating hot flashes generally incorporates a consultation with a homeopathic practitioner and the prescription of an individualized homeopathic remedy designed to address the symptoms reported by the study subject.

One randomized controlled trial, stratified for age, breast cancer stage, and tamoxifen use, showed no significant difference in hot flash activity over a one-year period (Jacobs, Herman, Heron, Olsen, & Vaughters, 2005).

Two observational studies of homeopathic treatment of hot flashes conducted at an outpatient homeopathic clinic in Glasgow, Scotland, reported improvement in hot flashes, but methodologic flaws were too numerous for the studies to be useful (Clover & Ratsey, 2002; Thompson & Reilly, 2003).

SOY SUPPLEMENTS

Soy supplements were provided to subjects in the form of capsules, tablets, powder, or beverage. Four double-blind controlled trials of soy supplements versus placebo for treatment of hot flashes in women with breast cancer, stratified for tamoxifen use, did not show a significant difference in hot flash symptoms between the placebo and soy supplement arms of the studies (MacGregor, Canney, Patterson, McDonald, & Paul, 2005; Nikander, Metsa-Heikkila, Ylikorkala, & Tiitinen, 2004; Quella et al., 2000; Van Patten, 2002).

One randomized controlled trial in men undergoing androgen deprivation therapy for prostate cancer did not show any significant improvement in hot flashes between men receiving soy isoflavones compared to those on placebo (Sharma et al., 2009).

Not Recommended for Practice

Interventions for which lack of effectiveness or harmfulness has been demonstrated by strong evidence from rigorously conducted studies, meta-analyses, or systematic reviews, or interventions where the costs, burden, or harms associated with the intervention exceed anticipated benefit

There are no interventions as of February 2010.

Expert Opinion

Low-risk interventions that are (1) consistent with sound clinical practice, (2) suggested by an expert in a peer-reviewed publication (journal or book chapter), and (3) for which limited evidence exists. An expert is an individual with peer-reviewed journal publications in the domain of interest.

There are no interventions as of February 2010.

Areas for Research

Methodologic Considerations

- Randomized trials should include arms of sufficient size to detect a statistical difference.
- Randomized trials should compare with a placebo instead of another strategy to decrease hot flashes.
- Trials should include samples that match for other characteristics such as treatment and age.
- Trials should be conducted with both men and women but not necessarily in the same trial.
- Measurements should address hot flash severity and the number of occurrences with objective measures.
- Cost analysis of interventions should be conducted.
- Feasibility of providing an intervention in general practice should be evaluated, especially for interventions that must be delivered by specialists.
- Studies should also consider the impact of the intervention on quality of life.
- Interventions should be implemented for a reasonable amount of time, and follow-up data should be collected for longer periods of time to better understand the durability of a response to an intervention.
- Studies with substantial attrition rates need to try to determine the source of attrition, especially if it is related to the intervention.
- For nonpharmacologic interventions, specific directions and details about the intervention need to be included so the study or intervention can genuinely be replicated.

Search Strategy

Computerized literature searching was done using the consolidated PICO terms as outlined below. No date limitation was used, and additional manual retrieval was done for key findings from the literature. The limitations of adults and English language were used. The final literature search was performed in February 2010.

Patient/Problem: Adult patients with prostate cancer or breast cancer with hot flashes

Intervention: All interventions, lifestyle, complementary therapies, supplements or naturopathy, or pharmacology

1. Lifestyle (exercise, diet, caffeine, alcoholic beverages, smoking, relaxation therapy)
2. Complementary therapies (hypnosis, biofeedback, meditation, yoga, deep breathing)
3. Supplements/naturopathy (Cimicifuga, black cohosh, isoflavones, soy, trifolium, red clover, naturopathy)
4. Pharmacologic (antidepressive agents, serotonin uptake inhibitors, clonidine, gabapentin, hormone replacement, megestrol acetate, medroxyprogesterone 17-acetate, venlafaxine, paroxetine, fluoxetine, citalopram, o-desmethylvenlafaxine, Effexor, paroxetine, Paxil® [GlaxoSmithKline], Prozac, Celexa® [Forest Pharmaceuticals], desvenlafaxine, Pristiq® [Pfizer], Neurontin® [Pfizer], hot flash drugs)

Comparison: None
Outcome: All
Limits: Adults and English language
Databases Used: PubMed, Ovid®, CINAHL®, EMBASE®, Cochrane Collaboration, Google™ Scholar

Definitions of terms and the complete evidence table are available at **www.ons.org/research/PEP**. Literature search completed through February 2010.

References

Agarwal, P., & Oefelein, M. (2005). Testosterone replacement therapy after primary treatment for prostate cancer. *Journal of Urology, 173,* 533–536. doi:10.1097/01.ju.0000143942.55896.64

Barton, D.L., Loprinzi, C.L., Quella, S.K., Sloan, J.A., Veeder, M.H., Egner, J.R., ... Novotny, P. (1998). Prospective evaluation of vitamin E for hot flashes in breast cancer survivors. *Journal of Clinical Oncology, 16,* 495–500.

Bertelli, G., Venturini, M., Del Mastro, L., Bergaglio, M., Sismondi, P., Biglia, N., ... Rosso, R. (2002). Intramuscular depot medroxyprogesterone versus oral megestrol for the control of postmenopausal hot flashes in breast cancer patients: A randomized study. *Annals of Oncology, 13,* 883–888.

Biglia, N., Kubatzki, F., Sgandurra, P., Ponzone, R., Marenco, D., Peano, E., & Sismondi, P. (2007). Mirtazapine for the treatment of hot flushes in breast cancer survivors: A prospective pilot trial. *Breast Journal, 13,* 490–495. doi:10.1111/j.1524-4741.2007.00470.x

Biglia, N., Sgandurra, P., Peano, E., Marenco, D., Moggio, G., Bounous, V., ... Sismondi, P. (2009). Nonhormonal treatment of hot flushes in breast cancer survivors: Gabapentin vs. vitamin E. *Climacteric, 12,* 310–318. doi:10.1080/13697130902736921

Biglia, N., Torta, R., Roagna, R., Maggiorotto, F., Cacciari, F., Ponzone, R., ... Sismondi, P. (2005). Evaluation of low-dose venlafaxine hydrochloride for the therapy of hot flushes in breast cancer survivors. *Maturitas, 52,* 78–85. doi:10.1016/j.maturitas.2005.01.001

Buijs, C., Mom, C.H., Willemse, P.H., Boezen, H.M., Maurer, J.M., Wymenga, A.N., ... Mourits, M.J. (2009). Venlafaxine versus clonidine for the treatment of hot flashes in breast cancer patients: A double-blind, randomized cross-over study. *Breast Cancer Research and Treatment, 115,* 573–580. doi:10.1007/s10549-008-0138-7

Carpenter, J.S., Storniolo, A.M., Johns, S., Monahan, P.O., Azzouz, F., Elam, J.L., ... Shelton, R.C. (2007). Randomized, double-blind, placebo-controlled crossover trials of venlafaxine for hot flashes after breast cancer. *Oncologist, 12,* 124–135. doi:10.1634/theoncologist.12-1-124

Carson, J.W., Carson, K.M., Porter, L.S., Keefe, F.J., & Seewaldt, V.L. (2009). Yoga of Awareness program for menopausal symptoms in breast cancer survivors: Results from a randomized trial. *Supportive Care in Cancer, 17,* 1301–1309. doi:10.1007/s00520-009-0587-5

Clover, A., & Ratsey, D. (2002). Homeopathic treatment of hot flushes: A pilot study. *Homeopathy, 91,* 75–79.

Deng, G., Vickers, A., Yeung, S., D'Andrea, G.M., Xiao, H., Heerdt, A.S., ... Cassileth, B. (2007). Randomized, controlled trial of acupuncture for the treatment of hot flashes in breast cancer patients. *Journal of Clinical Oncology, 25,* 5584–5590. doi:10.1200/JCO.2007.12.0774

Elkins, G., Marcus, J., Palamara, L., & Stearns, V. (2004). Can hypnosis reduce hot flashes in breast cancer survivors? A literature review. *American Journal of Clinical Hypnosis, 47,* 29–42.

Elkins, G., Marcus, J., Stearns, V., Perfect, M., Rajab, M.H., Ruud, C., ... Keith, T. (2008). Randomized trial of a hypnosis intervention for treatment of hot flashes among breast cancer survivors. *Journal of Clinical Oncology, 26,* 5022–5026. doi:10.1200/JCO.2008.16.6389

Elkins, G., Marcus, J., Stearns, V., & Rajab, M.H. (2007). Pilot evaluation of hypnosis for the treatment of hot flashes in breast cancer survivors. *Psycho-Oncology, 16,* 487–492. doi:10.1002/pon.1096

Fenlon, D.R., Corner, J.L., & Haviland, J.S. (2008). A randomized controlled trial of relaxation training to reduce hot flashes in women with primary breast cancer. *Journal of Pain and Symptom Management, 35,* 397–405. doi:10.1016/j.jpainsymman.2007.05.014

Filshie, J., Bolton, T., Browne, D., & Ashley, S. (2005). Acupuncture and self acupuncture for long-term treatment of vasomotor symptoms in cancer patients—Audit and treatment algorithm. *Acupuncture in Medicine, 23,* 171–180. doi:10.1136/aim.23.4.171

Frisk, J., Carlhall, S., Kallstrom, A.C., Lindh-Astrand, L., Malmstrom, A., & Hammar, M. (2008). Long-term follow-up of acupuncture and hormone therapy on hot flushes in women with breast cancer: A prospective, randomized, controlled multicenter trial. *Climacteric, 11,* 166–174. doi:10.1080/13697130801958709

Gerber, G.S., Zagaja, G.P., Ray, P.S., & Rukstalis, D.B. (2000). Transdermal estrogen in the treatment of hot flushes in men with prostate cancer. *Urology, 55,* 97–101. doi:10.1016/S0090-4295(99)00370-2

Goldberg, R.M., Loprinzi, C.L., O'Fallon, J.R., Veeder, M.H., Miser, A.W., Mailliard, J.A., ... Burnham, N.L. (1994). Transdermal clonidine for ameliorating tamoxifen-induced hot flashes. *Journal of Clinical Oncology, 12,* 155–158.

Goodwin, J.W., Green, S.J., Moinpour, C.M., Bearden, J.D., III, Giguere, J.K., Jiang, C.S., ... Albain, K.S. (2008). Phase III randomized placebo-controlled trial of two doses of megestrol acetate as treatment for menopausal symptoms in women with breast cancer: Southwest Oncology Group Study 9626. *Journal of Clinical Oncology, 26,* 1650–1656. doi:10.1200/JCO.2006.10.6179

Hammar, M., Frisk, J., Grimås, O., Höök, M., Spetz, A.C., & Wyon, Y. (1999). Acupuncture treatment of vasomotor symptoms in men with prostatic carcinoma: A pilot study. *Journal of Urology, 161,* 853–856. doi:10.1016/S0022-5347(01)61789-0

Harding, C., Harris, A., & Chadwick, D. (2008). Auricular acupuncture: A novel treatment for vasomotor symptoms associated with luteinizing-hormone releasing hormone agonist treatment for prostate cancer. *British Journal of Urology International, 103,* 186–190. doi:10.1111/j.1464-410X.2008.07884.x

Hervik, J., & Mjåland, J. (2009). Acupuncture for the treatment of hot flashes in breast cancer patients, a randomized, controlled trial. *Breast Cancer Research and Treatment, 116,* 311–316. doi:10.1007/s10549-008-0210-3

Jacobs, J., Herman, P., Heron, K., Olsen, S., & Vaughters, L. (2005). Homeopathy for menopausal symptoms in breast cancer survivors: A preliminary randomized controlled trial. *Journal of Alternative and Complementary Medicine, 11,* 21–27. doi:10.1089/acm.2005.11.21

Jacobson, J.S., Troxel, A.B., Evans, J., Klaus, L., Vahdat, L., Kinne, D., ... Grann, V.R. (2001). Randomized trial of black cohosh for the treatment of hot flashes among women with a history of breast cancer. *Journal of Clinical Oncology, 19,* 2739–2745. Retrieved from http://jco.ascopubs.org/cgi/reprint/19/10/2739

Kelly, C., Juurlink, D., Gomes, T., Duong-Hua, M., Pritchard, K., Austin, P., & Paszat, L. (2010). Selective serotonin reuptake inhibitors and breast cancer mortality in women. *BMJ, 340,* c693. doi:10.1136/bmj.c693

Kimmick, G.G., Lovato, J., McQuellon, R., Robinson, E., & Muss, H.B. (2006). Randomized, double-blind, placebo-controlled, crossover study of sertraline (Zoloft) for the treatment of hot flashes in women with early stage breast cancer taking tamoxifen. *Breast Journal, 12,* 114–122. doi:10.1111/j.1075-122X.2006.00218.x

Kroiss, R., Fentiman, I.S., Helmond, F.A., Rymer, J., Foidart, J.M., Bundred, N., ... Kubista, E. (2005). The effect of tibolone in postmenopausal women receiving tamoxifen after surgery for breast cancer: A randomised, double-blind, placebo-controlled trial. *BJOG, 112,* 228–233. doi:10.1111/j.1471-0528.2004.00309.x

Lipov, E.G., Joshi, J.R., Sanders, S., Wilcox, K., Lipov, S., Xie, H., ... Slavin, K. (2008). Effects of stellate-ganglion block on hot flushes and night awakenings in survivors of breast cancer: A pilot study. *Lancet Oncology, 9,* 523–532. doi:10.1016/S1470-2045(08)70131-1

Loibl, S., Schwedler, K., von Minckwitz, G., Strohmeier, R., Mehta, K.M., & Kaufmann, M. (2007). Venlafaxine is superior to clonidine as treatment of hot flashes in breast cancer patients—A double-blind, randomized study. *Annals of Oncology, 18,* 689–693. doi:10.1093/annonc/mdl478

Loprinzi, C.L., Sloan, J.A., Perez, E.A., Quella, S.K., Stella, P.J., Mailliard, J.A., ... Rummans, T.A. (2002). Phase III evaluation of fluoxetine for treatment of hot flashes. *Journal of Clinical Oncology, 20,* 1578–1583. doi:10.1200/JCO.20.6.1578

Loprinzi, C.L., Kugler, J.W., Sloan, J.A., Mailliard, J.A., LaVasseur, B.I., Barton, D.L., ... Christensen, B.J. (2000). Venlafaxine in management of hot flashes in survivors of breast cancer: A randomised controlled trial. *Lancet, 356,* 2059–2063. doi:10.1016/S0140-6736(00)03403-6

Loprinzi, C.L., Michalak, J.C., Quella, S.K., O'Fallon, J.R., Hatfield, A.K., Nelimark, R.A., ... Oesterling, J.E. (1994). Megestrol acetate for the prevention of hot flashes. *New England Journal of Medicine, 331,* 347–352. doi:10.1056/NEJM199408113310602

Loprinzi, C.L., Sloan, J., Stearns, V., Slack, R., Iyengar, M., Diekmann, B., ... Novotny, P. (2009). Newer antidepressants and gabapentin for hot flashes: An individual patient pooled analysis. *Journal of Clinical Oncology, 27,* 2831–2837. doi:10.1200/JCO.2008.19.6253

MacGregor, C.A., Canney, P.A., Patterson, G., McDonald, R., & Paul, J. (2005). A randomised double-blind controlled trial of oral soy supplements versus placebo for treatment of menopausal symptoms in patients with early breast cancer. *European Journal of Cancer, 41,* 708–714. doi:10.1016/j.ejca.2005.01.005

Muñoz, G.H., & Pluchino, S. (2003). Cimicifuga racemosa for the treatment of hot flushes in women surviving breast cancer. *Maturitas, 44*(Suppl. 1), S59–S65. doi:10.1016/S0378-5122(02)00349-3

National Cancer Institute. (n.d.). Dictionary of cancer terms: Black cohosh. Retrieved from http://www.cancer.gov/dictionary/?CdrID=321355

Nedstrand, E., Wijma, K., Wyon, Y., & Hammar, M. (2005). Vasomotor symptoms decrease in women with breast cancer randomized to treatment with applied relaxation or electro-acupuncture: A preliminary study. *Climacteric, 8,* 243–250. doi:10.1080/13697130500118050

Nikander, E., Metsa-Heikkila, M., Ylikorkala, O., & Tiitinen, A. (2004). Effects of phytoestrogens on bone turn-over in postmenopausal women with a history of breast cancer. *Journal of Clinical Endocrinology and Metabolism, 89,* 1207–1212.

Pandya, K.J., Morrow, G.R., Roscoe, J.A., Zhao, H., Hickok, J.T., Pajon, E., … Flynn, P.J. (2005). Gabapentin for hot flashes in 420 women with breast cancer: A randomised double-blind placebo-controlled trial. *Lancet, 366,* 818–824. doi:10.1016/S0140-6736(05)67215-7

Pandya, K.J., Raubertas, R.F., Flynn, P.J., Hynes, H.E., Rosenbluth, R.J., Kirshner, J.J., … Morrow, G.R. (2000). Oral clonidine in postmenopausal patients with breast cancer experiencing tamoxifen-induced hot flashes: A University of Rochester Cancer Center community clinical oncology program study. *Annals of Internal Medicine, 132,* 788–793.

Pockaj, B.A., Gallagher, J.G., Loprinzi, C.L., Stella, P.J., Barton, D.L., Sloan, J.A., … Fauq, A.H. (2006). Phase III double-blind, randomized, placebo-controlled crossover trial of black cohosh in the management of hot flashes: NCCTG trial N01CC1. *Journal of Clinical Oncology, 24,* 2836–2841. doi:10.1200/JCO.2005.05.4296

Quella, S.K., Loprinzi, C.L., Barton, D.L., Knost, J.A., Sloan, J.A., LaVasseur, B.I., … Novotny, P.J. (2000). Evaluation of soy phytoestrogens for the treatment of hot flashes in breast cancer survivors: A North Central Cancer Treatment group trial. *Journal of Clinical Oncology, 18,* 1068–1074. Retrieved from http://jco.ascopubs.org/content/18/5/1068.long

Schover, L.R., Jenkins, R., Sui, D., Adams, J.H., Marion, M.S., & Jackson, K.E. (2006). Randomized trial of peer counseling on reproductive health in African American breast cancer survivors. *Journal of Clinical Oncology, 24,* 1620–1626. doi:10.1200/JCO.2005.04.7159

Sharma, P., Wisniewski, A., Braga-Basaria, M., Xu, X., Yep, M., Denmeade, S., … Basaria, S. (2009). Lack of an effect of high dose isoflavones in men with prostate cancer undergoing androgen deprivation therapy. *Journal of Urology, 182,* 2265–2272. doi:10.1016/j.juro.2009.07.030

Stearns, V., Slack, R., Greep, N., Henry-Tilman, R., Osborne, M., Bunnell, C., … Isaacs, C. (2005). Paroxetine is an effective treatment for hot flashes: Results from a prospective randomized clinical trial. *Journal of Clinical Oncology, 23,* 6919–6930. doi:10.1200/JCO.2005.10.081

Thompson, E.A., & Reilly, D. (2003). The homeopathic approach to the treatment of symptoms of oestrogen withdrawal in breast cancer patients: A prospective observational study. *Homeopathy, 92,* 131–134.

Towlerton, G., O'Brien, M., & Duncan, A. (1999). Acupuncture in the control of vasomotor symptoms caused by tamoxifen. *Palliative Medicine, 13,* 445. doi:10.1177/026921639901300516

Van Patten, C.L. (2002). Effect of soy phytoestrogens on hot flashes in postmenopausal women with breast cancer: A randomized, controlled clinical trial. *Journal of Clinical Oncology, 20,* 1449–1455. doi:10.1200/JCO.20.6.1449

Walker, E.M., Rodriguez, A.I., Kohn, B., Ball, R.M., Pegg, J., Pocock, J.R., … Levine, R.A. (2010). Acupuncture versus venlafaxine for the management of vasomotor symptoms in patients with hormone receptor-positive breast cancer: A randomized controlled trial. *Journal of Clinical Oncology, 28,* 634–640. doi:10.1200/JCO.2009.23.5150

Younus, J., Simpson, I., Collins, A., & Wang, X. (2003). Mind control of menopause. *Women's Health Issues, 13,* 74–78. doi:10.1016/S1049-3867(02)00196-2

CHAPTER **4**

Radiodermatitis

Editor, Tara Baney, RN, MS, ANP-BC, AOCN®

Problem

Radiodermatitis, also known as *radiation dermatitis* or *radiation skin reaction*, is associated with the integumentary system's response to the planned exposure of ionizing radiation, which causes depletion of stem cells from the basal layer of the epidermis. Radiation repeatedly interrupts the repopulation of the skin's cells, weakening the integrity of the skin within the treatment field (Bolderston et al., 2006). The severity of radiodermatitis is affected by many factors related to the host, treatment modality, and location of therapy. A reaction can affect quality of life and outcomes if it becomes a source of significant pain and discomfort, limits daily activities, or causes treatment interruptions (Aistars, 2006). If radiodermatitis is severe enough, treatment cessation is often temporarily or permanently necessary.

Incidence

In developed countries such as the United States, Canada, European nations, and Australia, at least 50% of all patients with cancer will receive radiotherapy at some stage during the illness trajectory (Bernier et al., 2008). As a result, a substantial number of people with cancer can expect to develop radiation dermatitis. Even with the benefits of contemporary techniques for sparing the skin, as many as 95% of patients experience some degree of reaction of the integumentary system (De Conno, Ventafridda, & Saita, 1991; King, Nail, Kreamer, Strohl, & Johnson, 1985; Porock & Kristjanson, 1999). The exact incidence of radiation dermatitis associated with newer technology and treatment modalities is not fully understood (Bernier et al., 2008; Hymes, Strom, & Fife, 2006; Pignol et al., 2008).

Prevention

Skin reactions may be expected to occur as a result of radiation entering and exiting the skin or being deposited at the surface of the skin (Khan, 2003; Porock &

Kristjanson, 1999). Prevention is often considered as the complete avoidance of any detrimental skin changes; however, in the context of skin reactions, prevention is about delaying the onset and preventing the progression or deterioration to higher grades of dermatitis (Primavera et al., 2006). Evidence and consensus are limited to support the use of products for the prevention of acute radiation skin reactions (Bolderston et al., 2006; Röper, Kaisig, Auer, Mergen, & Molls, 2004).

Patient variability expressed in normal tissue reactions to radiation therapy can be explained by the interplay of treatment-related factors (treatment field location and volume, total dose and duration of treatment, individual fraction size, type of energy, and the use of bolus or tissue equivalent material), genetic factors, and personal factors (areas of skin friction, existing compromised skin integrity, comorbid conditions, nutritional status, age, race, ethnicity, drug therapies, sun exposure, and smoking) (Ryan et al., 2007). Consideration of this interplay could be useful in identifying individuals with risk factors affecting the degree of skin reactions (Porock, 2002).

General supportive measures for acute radiation dermatitis include washing with mild soap, keeping the treated area clean and dry, wearing loose-fitting clothes made of natural fibers, and protecting the radiation field from further physical or chemical irritants, such as ultraviolet light (Omidvari et al., 2007).

Survivorship and Late Effects

Radiation treatment not only causes radiodermatitis during treatment, with early resolution of the acute reaction within weeks of completing treatment, but also is associated with several risks or problems facing the patient following treatment. This can include radiation recall as well as late effects such as hypo- and hyperpigmentation, telangiectasia (visible spider-like veins), photosensitivity, xerosis (dry skin), atrophy, skin fibrosis, and delayed wound healing following surgical treatment in the radiation treatment field (Hymes et al., 2006).

Radiation Recall Dermatitis

Radiation recall is an acute reaction and inflammation in response to a systemic drug. A hypothesis is that the cells within the radiation treatment field "remember" the radiation skin reaction and are stimulated again when exposed to a sensitizing drug or that the cells are genetically mutated and are unable to tolerate the exposure of that drug. Another theory is a drug sensitivity or hypersensitivity in an immunocompromised host (Azria et al., 2005; Caloglu et al., 2007). The recall reaction appears as dermatitis ranging from mild erythema to a severe pruritic scaly rash (Kodym et al., 2005). It is typically seen in the radiation treatment field but can also occur in other tissues, including organs, muscle, and oral mucosa. A radiation recall reaction may occur months to years following the radiotherapy treatment but will also appear within days to a couple of months following the introduction of a triggering agent. Triggering agents can include chemotherapy drugs (e.g., methotrexate, 5-fluorouracil, alkylating agents, anthracyclines, taxanes, gemcitabine), as well as antimicrobials, immunotherapy drugs, and hormonal agents (Thomas & Stea, 2002; Yeo & Johnson, 2000).

Late Effects

Late effects may appear months to years after exposure to radiation treatment. Pigmentation changes result from damage to melanocytes, and telangiectasia results from damage and stretching of the small blood vessels possibly associated with moist desquamation reactions during treatment (O'Sullivan & Levin, 2003). Fibrosis is a result of alterations in the inflammatory, proliferative, and tissue remodeling phases of wound healing following radiation dermatitis. DNA damage and the subsequent cytokine cascade results in excessive extracellular matrix and collagen being deposited in the wound. This can lead to reduced tissue flexibility, atrophy, reduced tissue strength, strictures, and reduced range of motion. The patient is also at increased risk for delayed wound healing, dehiscence, fistulas, skin flap failures, and other complications following surgical procedures within the radiation treatment field (Bentzen, 2006; McQuestion, 2010).

Although late effects have been well described in the literature, both the prevention and management of late radiation skin effects have a paucity of available research. Anecdotally, acute radiation skin effects seem to have been reduced across patient populations with the implementation of intensity-modulated radiation therapy (IMRT). Only one study has been published showing a reduction in the severity and duration of moist desquamation (grade 2 and 3) with the use of IMRT in the treatment of breast cancer (Freedman et al., 2009). Whether that translates into a reduction in late radiation skin effects has yet to be determined. Furthermore, literature is limited to support interventions for late effects management. Only one study addresses the use of mechanical massage for treating radiation-induced skin fibrosis in women with breast cancer (Bourgeois, Gourgou, Kramar, Lagarde, & Guillot, 2008). Future research needs to address the prevention and management of late or chronic skin changes resulting from radiation treatment.

Assessment and Clinical Measurement Tools

Commonly used grading or scoring tools for the assessment and documentation of radiodermatitis include the Radiation Therapy Oncology Group (RTOG) Acute Radiation Morbidity Scoring Criteria (Cox, Stetz, & Pajak, 1995), the RTOG/EORTC (European Organization for Research and Treatment of Cancer) Late Radiation Morbidity Scoring Scheme (Cox et al., 1995), the National Cancer Institute (NCI) Cancer Therapy Evaluation Program (2010) *Common Terminology Criteria for Adverse Events*, the Skin Toxicity Assessment Tool (Berthelet et al., 2004), the Oncology Nursing Society (Catlin-Huth, Pollock, & Haas, 2002) Acute Skin Toxicity Scale using NCI's common toxicity criteria, and the Radiation-Induced Skin Reaction Assessment Scale (Noble-Adams, 1999a, 1999b).

Each assessment tool can be used to identify grades or degrees of skin reactions, including erythema, dry desquamation, and moist desquamation. The majority of tools are assessments that the practitioner or observer completes and, thus, do not capture the symptoms or impact of the skin reaction (see Table 4-1). Skin should be assessed as a baseline prior to the initiation of treatment and, at a minimum, at weekly review appointments. The skin assessment should include changes in color, appearance of patchy dry desquamation, patchy or confluent moist desquamation, presence or absence of drainage, presence or absence of odor, and signs of infection. The patient's symptoms, such as the sensation of dryness, pruritus, or pain, must also be taken into account. The distress and impact associated with the radiodermatitis on quality of life, daily living, self-care ability, and financial impact of caring for the skin reaction are also important areas of assessment.

Table 4-1. Clinical Measurement Tools for Radiodermatitis

Tool	Description	Benefits and/or Limitations
Radiation Therapy Oncology Group Acute Radiation Morbidity Scoring Criteria (1985) (Cox et al., 1995)	Assesses intensity or severity of reaction Ordinal scale 0–4	No reliability or validity data published Observation of physical changes Does not address symptoms or patient perspective Commonly used in clinical trials
Radiation Therapy Oncology Group/ European Organization for Research and Treatment of Cancer toxicity criteria (Cox et al., 1995)	Assesses late complications Ordinal scale 1–4 Acute: less than 90 days after first treatment Late: after day 90 Also assesses for fibrosis, induration, skin contracture, and necrosis	No reliability or validity data published Observation of physical changes Does not address symptoms or patient perspective
Common Terminology Criteria for Adverse Events [v.4.03] Version 2.0 incorporated into the Oncology Nursing Society *Radiation Therapy Patient Care Record* for Radiation Dermatitis by Site Group (Catlin-Huth et al., 2002)	Adverse events reporting tool Severity scale Rash: dermatitis associated with radiation Ordinal scale 0–5 Grades of desquamation	No reliability or validity data published Observation of physical changes Does not address symptoms or patient perspective
Skin Toxicity Assessment Tool (known as STAT) (Berthelet et al., 2004)	Three areas of assessment Patient and treatment factors affecting incidence and intensity of radiodermatitis Objective scoring of grades of desquamation Patient symptoms	Preliminary reliability and validity results reported (Berthelet et al., 2004) Easy to use in the clinical setting Quickly administered

(Continued on next page)

Table 4-1. Clinical Measurement Tools for Radiodermatitis *(Continued)*		
Tool	**Description**	**Benefits and/or Limitations**
Radiation-Induced Skin Reaction Assessment Scale (known as RISRAS) (Noble-Adams, 1999a, 1999b)	Weighted categories (e.g., moist desquamation weighted higher than dry desquamation) for overall score that incorporates effect on patient Symptom scale (e.g., tenderness, itching, burning, warmth, effect on activity) Observer assessment (e.g., erythema, dry desquamation, moist desquamation, necrosis)	Nursing assessment tool Objective observer assessment and patient's perspective of symptoms Reliability and validity scores have been reported. Has not been widely used in practice or research

References

Aistars, J. (2006). The validity of skin care protocols followed by women with breast cancer receiving external radiation. *Clinical Journal of Oncology Nursing, 10,* 487–492. doi:10.1188/06.CJON.487-492

Azria, D., Magné, N., Souhair, A., Castadot, P., Culine, S., Ychou, M., … Ozsahin, M. (2005). Radiation recall: A well recognized but neglected phenomenon. *Cancer Treatment Reviews, 31,* 555–570. doi:10.1016/j.ctrv.2005.07.008

Bentzen, S.M. (2006). Preventing or reducing late side effects of radiation therapy: Radiobiology meets molecular pathology. *Nature Reviews Cancer, 6,* 702–713. doi:10.1038/nrc1950

Bernier, J., Bonner, J., Vermorken, J.B., Bensadoun, R.-J., Dummer, R., Giralt, J., … Ang, K.K. (2008). Consensus guidelines for the management of radiation dermatitis and coexisting acne-like rash in patients receiving radiotherapy plus EGFR inhibitors for the treatment of squamous cell carcinoma of the head and neck. *Annals of Oncology, 19,* 142–149. doi:10.1093/annonc/mdm400

Berthelet, E., Truong, P.T., Musso, K., Grant, V., Kwan, W., Moravan, V., … Olivotto, I.A. (2004). Preliminary reliability and validity testing of a new skin toxicity assessment tool (STAT) in breast cancer patients undergoing radiotherapy. *American Journal of Clinical Oncology, 27,* 626–631.

Bolderston, A., Lloyd, N.S., Wong, R.K.S., Holden, L., Robb-Blenderman, L., & Supportive Care Guidelines Group. (2006). *The prevention and management of acute skin reactions related to radiation therapy: A clinical practice guideline* (Practice Guidelines Report #13-7). Toronto, Ontario, Canada: Cancer Care Ontario.

Bourgeois, J.F., Gourgou, S., Kramar, A., Lagarde, J.M., & Guillot, B. (2008). A randomized, prospective study using the LPG technique in treating radiation-induced skin fibrosis: Clinical and profilometric analysis. *Skin Research and Technology, 14,* 71–76. doi:10.1111/j.1600-0846.2007.00263.x

Caloglu, M., Yurut-Caloglu, V., Cosar-Alas, R., Saynak, M., Karagol, H., & Uzal, C. (2007). An ambiguous phenomenon of radiation and drugs: Recall reactions. *Onkologie, 30,* 209–214. doi:10.1159/000099632

Catlin-Huth, C., Pollock, V., & Haas, M. (Eds.). (2002). *Radiation therapy patient care record: A tool for documenting nursing care* (2nd ed.). Pittsburgh, PA: Oncology Nursing Society.

Cox, J.D., Stetz, B.S., & Pajak, T.F. (1995). Toxicity criteria of the Radiation Therapy Oncology Group (RTOG) and the European Organization for Research and Treatment of Cancer (EORTC). *International Journal of Radiation Oncology, Biology, Physics, 31,* 1341–1346. doi:10.1016/0360-3016(95)00060-C

De Conno, F., Ventafridda, V., & Saita, L. (1991). Skin problems in advanced and terminal cancer patients. *Journal of Pain and Symptom Management, 6,* 247–256. doi:10.1016/0885-3924(91)90015-V

Freedman, G.M., Li, T., Nicolaou, N., Chen, Y., Ma, C.C.-M., & Anderson, P.R. (2009). Breast intensity-modulated radiation therapy reduces time spent with acute dermatitis for women of all breast sizes during radiation. *International Journal of Radiation Oncology, Biology, Physics, 74,* 689–694. doi:10.1016/j.ijrobp.2008.08.071

Hymes, S.R., Strom, E.A., & Fife, C. (2006). Radiation dermatitis: Clinical presentation, pathophysiology, and treatment. *Journal of the American Academy of Dermatology, 54,* 28–46. doi:10.1016/j.jaad.2005.08.054

Khan, F.M. (2003). *The physics of radiation therapy* (3rd ed.). Philadelphia, PA: Lippincott Williams & Wilkins.

King, K.B., Nail, L.M., Kreamer, K., Strohl, R.A., & Johnson, J.E. (1985). Patients' descriptions of the experience of receiving radiation therapy. *Oncology Nursing Forum, 12*(4), 55–61.

Kodym, E., Kalinska, R., Ehringfeld, C., Sterbik-Lamina, A., Kodym, R., & Hohenberg, G. (2005). Frequency of radiation recall dermatitis in adult cancer patients. *Onkologie, 28,* 18–21. doi:10.1159/000082175

McQuestion, M. (2010). Radiation-induced skin reactions. In M.L. Haas & G.J. Moore-Higgs (Eds.), *Principles of skin care and the oncology patient* (pp. 115–140). Pittsburgh, PA: Oncology Nursing Society.

National Cancer Institute Cancer Therapy Evaluation Program. (2010). *Common terminology criteria for adverse events* [v.4.03]. Retrieved from http://evs.nci.nih.gov/ftp1/CTCAE/CTCAE_4.03_2010-06-14_QuickReference_5x7.pdf

Noble-Adams, R. (1999a). Radiation-induced skin reactions 2: Development of a measurement tool. *British Journal of Nursing, 8,* 1208–1211.

Noble-Adams, R. (1999b). Radiation-induced skin reactions 3: Evaluating the RISRAS. *British Journal of Nursing, 8,* 1305–1312.

Omidvari, S., Saboori, H., Mohammadianpanah, M., Mosalaei, A., Ahmadloo, N., Mosleh-Shirazi, M.A., … Namaz, S. (2007). Topical betamethasone for prevention of radiation dermatitis. *Indian Journal of Dermatology, Venereology and Leprology, 73,* 209–214.

O'Sullivan, B., & Levin, W. (2003). Late radiation-related fibrosis: Pathogenesis, manifestations, and current management. *Seminars in Radiation Oncology, 13,* 274–289. doi:10.1016/S1053-4296(03)00037-7

Pignol, J.P., Olivotto, I., Rakovitch, E., Gardner, S., Sixel, K., Beckham, W., … Paszat, L. (2008). A multicenter randomized trial of breast intensity-modulated radiation therapy to reduce acute radiation dermatitis. *Journal of Clinical Oncology, 26,* 2085–2092. doi:10.1200/JCO.2007.15.2488

Porock, D. (2002). Factors influencing the severity of radiation skin and oral mucosal reactions: Development of a conceptual framework. *European Journal of Cancer Care, 11,* 33–43. doi:10.1111/j.1365-2354.2002.00287.x

Porock, D., & Kristjanson, L. (1999). Skin reactions during radiotherapy for breast cancer: The use and impact of topical agents and dressings. *European Journal of Cancer Care, 8,* 143–153. doi:10.1046/j.1365-2354.1999.00153.x

Röper, B., Kaisig, D., Auer, F., Mergen, E., & Molls, M. (2004). Theta-Cream versus Bepanthol lotion in breast cancer patients under radiotherapy. *Strahlentherapie und Onkologie, 180,* 315–322. doi:10.1007/s00066-004-1174-9

Ryan, J.L., Bole, C., Hickok, J.T., Figueroa-Mosely, C., Colman, L., Khanna, R.C., … Morrow, G.R. (2007). Post-treatment skin reactions reported by cancer patients differ by race, not by treatment or expectations. *British Journal of Cancer, 97,* 14–21. doi:10.1038/sj.bjc.6603842

Thomas, R., & Stea, B. (2002). Radiation recall dermatitis from high-dose interferon alfa-2b. *Journal of Clinical Oncology, 20,* 355–357. Retrieved from http://jco.ascopubs.org/content/20/1/355.full.pdf+html

Yeo, W., & Johnson, P.J. (2000). Radiation-recall skin disorders associated with the use of antineoplastic drugs: Pathogenesis, prevalence, and management. *American Journal of Clinical Dermatology, 1,* 113–116.

Case Study

S.R. is a 62-year-old man who was recently diagnosed with a T3N2M0 squamous cell carcinoma at the base of his tongue. He underwent combined modality treatment, including IMRT for 70 Gy (7,000 cGy) in 35 daily fractions, Monday to Friday for 7 weeks, plus 3 cycles of high-dose cisplatin 100 mg/m^2 at weeks 1, 4, and 7.

Past medical history included hypertension, gastroesophageal reflux disease, and a recent onset of non–insulin-dependent diabetes mellitus (NIDDM). Medications included atenolol 50 mg daily, rabeprazole 20 mg twice daily, and metformin 1,000 mg twice daily. S.R. was also morbidly obese (body mass index greater than 40), with a weight of 287 lbs for his height of 5 feet 9 inches. He indicated he ate a diet mostly of pasta and meats with few fruits and vegetables. He also smoked one pack of cigarettes a day for 35 years and indicated that he consumed 24 beers every weekend while at the cottage. S.R. quit smoking after receiving his diagnosis of cancer.

The nurse identified several risk factors related to a potential increased severity of skin reaction during treatment, including receiving radiation treatment to the head and neck area, a large volume of tissue being irradiated (primary tumor plus bilateral neck), the inclusion of chemotherapy in the treatment protocol, and a treatment duration of seven weeks with the use of electrons to the neck nodes. Additionally, S.R. had significant skin folds in the neck because of obesity, and he had NIDDM, poor nutrition, and regular sun exposure related to his cottage and outdoor activities.

From the onset of treatment, S.R. was advised to continue washing his face and neck with a mild soap and water while maintaining his usual hygiene pattern. He was also told to use a moisturizer or cream such as hyaluronic acid or calendula cream across the treatment field until he experienced any skin breakdown.

When S.R. reached 36 Gy (3,600 cGy 18 fractions) of radiation dose, he was experiencing mild erythema in the treatment field (RTOG 1). By 44 Gy (22 fractions), the skin reaction had increased to moderate erythema over the treatment field with patchy dry desquamation in a line across the lower jaw under the chin (RTOG 2).

At 56 Gy (28 fractions), he had bright erythema with dry desquamation in a larger area across the anterior and lateral aspects of his neck. S.R. was advised to continue to wash the area and to use saline soaks over the dry desquamation to remove dry scaling tissue and provide comfort through cooling and soothing the tissue (no open oozing areas). He was also advised to continue to generously apply the hyaluronic acid or calendula cream throughout the day and at bedtime.

Near the completion of treatment at 62 Gy (31 fractions), S.R. was experiencing confluent moist desquamation over the neck skin folds as well as the anterior chest (RTOG 3). Although limited evidence is available for the use of various products for the management of moist desquamation, the institutional standard based on expert opinion (see the *Expert Opinion* section in the PEP Resource) would suggest using dressings to protect the wound, reduce pain, and provide comfort by reducing friction and trauma with exposure. Options might include a silver leaf dressing, Mepilex® (Mölnlycke Health Care), or other nonstick dressings, changed once or twice daily, as needed. Dressings would be removed prior to treatment and then reapplied after treatment before the patient goes home. A referral to a wound care specialist within the organization or the community could be made.

During the last review appointment as S.R. was completing his seven weeks of radiation, the nurse discussed expectations, pattern, and pace of healing of the radiodermatitis reaction. He was also advised of sun sense and skin protection following treatment. He was advised that healing would take place over the next two to four weeks once the radiation treatment was complete. The nurse suggested that he continue with the current end-of-treatment skin care regimen and to compare changes on a weekly basis so improvements would be visible, rather than day to day where only subtle improvements may occur. By the second week after treatment, the moist desquamation was expected to heal with new pink tissue replacing the open desquamated areas. By week three, the skin tone would be returning to normal, whereby S.R. would still be able to see the outline of the treatment field but it would be less visible to other people. By week four, the skin was expected to heal and return to the normal skin tone.

During a follow-up appointment two weeks after treatment, S.R.'s skin was healing well with no areas of moist desquamation. He was to resume the use of hyaluronic acid or calendula cream as a moisturizer as the skin continues to heal.

Radiodermatitis

AUTHORS
Tara Baney, RN, MS, ANP-BC, AOCN®, Maurene Mcquestion, RN, BScN, MSc, CON(C),
Kathleen Bell, RN, MSN, OCN®, Susan Bruce, RN, MSN, OCN®,
Deborah Feight, RN, MSN, CNS, AOCN®, Linda Weis-Smith, RN, OCN®, and
Marilyn Haas, PhD, RN, CNS, ANP-C
LIBRARIAN: Mark Vrabel, MLS, AHIP, ELS
ONS STAFF: Margaret Irwin, PhD, RN, MN

What interventions are effective in preventing and treating radiation dermatitis?

Recommended for Practice

Interventions for which effectiveness has been demonstrated by strong evidence from rigorously conducted studies, meta-analyses, or systematic reviews and for which expectation of harms is small compared with the benefits

INTENSITY-MODULATED RADIATION THERAPY

Reduced skin toxicity during radiation therapy in patients receiving intensity-modulated radiation therapy (IMRT) versus conventional radiation therapy was demonstrated in three studies, using the *Common Terminology Criteria for Adverse Events*. Freedman et al. (2009) compared results between 399 women treated with IMRT and 405 women treated with conventional radiation treatment for breast cancer. In all breast size groupings, the IMRT group had significantly fewer patients who developed grade 2 or higher skin toxicity ($p \leq 0.0004$) and less time spent with grade 2 or 3 dermatitis ($p < 0.00001$) (Freedman et al., 2009). Using the National Cancer Institute (NCI) *Common Toxicity Criteria* (CTC), Pignol et al. (2008) looked at skin reactions and pain in women with early-stage breast cancer in 170 treated with IMRT versus 161 treated with conventional therapy. This study found that a lower proportion of patients treated with IMRT experienced moist desquamation during treatment and up to six weeks after radiation treatment, compared to conventional therapy ($p = 0.002$). Multivariate analysis demonstrated that IMRT ($p = 0.003$) and smaller breast size ($p = 0.001$) were associated with decreased risk of moist desquamation (Pignol et al., 2008).

In 2006, Freedman et al. looked at 73 women with breast cancer who received IMRT compared to 60 historical controls treated with conventional therapy. Acute skin toxicity was measured with the NCI CTC scoring; erythema and desquamation were also graded. This study found that 21% of IMRT patients developed moist desquamation, compared to 38% in the conventional group ($p = 0.0001$). The use of IMRT ($p = 0.001$) and breast size ($p < 0.0001$) were the only significant predictors of moist desquamation (Freedman et al., 2006).

USUAL HYGIENE PRACTICES: WASHING AND USE OF DEODORANT

Traditionally, washing the skin and using deodorants during radiation therapy have been controversial (McQuestion, 2010). Gentle skin and hair washing should be unrestricted in patients receiving radiation therapy, mild pH-neutral soap use is acceptable, and personal hygiene habits should be encouraged (Bernier et al., 2008; Bolderston et al., 2006).

Three research studies demonstrated that washing the skin in the irradiated field with either mild soap and water or water alone did not result in increased skin toxicity. A sample of 95 females treated with radiation therapy for breast cancer who were randomized to washing had reduction in pruritus compared to the group who did not wash (p > 0.05). No differences were observed between groups in other measures, and researchers concluded that findings supported allowing patients to wash during radiation therapy (Campbell & Illingworth, 1992).

Roy, Fortin, and Larochelle (2001) randomized 99 patients with breast cancer who were receiving adjuvant radiation therapy to either washing or no washing of the treatment field. Subjects who washed had lower overall maximum skin toxicity scores according to Radiation Therapy Oncology Group (RTOG) scoring (p = 0.04). No significant differences between groups were reported in time to maximal toxicity or erythema. However, the incidence of dry and moist desquamation was higher in the group that did not wash. The study concluded that washing skin that is undergoing radiation did not result in increased toxicity.

Westbury, Hines, Hawkes, Ashley, and Brada (2000) studied 107 patients who were receiving cranial radiotherapy to determine whether the patients' usual scalp care practice affects skin side effects of radiation therapy. Subjects ranged in age from 16–81 years. Pain, pruritus, skin reaction, and distress of changing hygiene practices were evaluated. Using the RTOG scale, an increase in severity of skin reactions during radiation therapy was not observed in the hair washing group. The group that did not wash experienced distress in change of hygiene practices.

Finally, a study showed that patients' use of their total usual skin care regimen did not result in any increased severity of skin reactions during and after completion of radiation therapy. Meegan and Haycocks (1997) reported findings in two groups of patients: 94 patients using warm water only and avoiding use of all lotions, soaps, and deodorants in the treatment field and 64 patients who continued with no restrictions of their normal skin care practices. The investigators observed no differences in the severity of skin reactions, and patient self-scoring of the severity of skin reactions was consistently higher in the unrestricted group.

Controversy regarding the use of deodorants has existed because of concerns about the direct effect on the skin and the potential effect on the surface dose of radiation therapy. One clinical study and one nonclinical study were found that addressed these concerns. In a study by Théberge, Harel, and Dagnault (2009), 84 female patients with breast cancer were randomly assigned to aluminum-free deodorant versus no deodorant after stratification by presence of axillary radiation therapy and adjuvant chemotherapy. The no-deodorant group had higher prevalence of moist desquamation (p = 0.003), more severe axillary (p = 0.019) and breast (p = 0.049) radiodermatitis, and higher prevalence of moderate to severe pain (p = 0.031).

Burch, Parker, Vann, and Arazie (1997) examined skin surface doses with 15 different products, including deodorants, powders, and creams, using an ionization chamber with large and small field sizes. They found very little difference in surface doses among the products examined (Burch et al., 1997). These findings lend further support to clinical findings regarding the acceptability of deodorant and usual skin care practice use.

Likely to Be Effective

Interventions for which effectiveness has been demonstrated by supportive evidence from a single rigorously conducted controlled trial, consistent supportive evidence from well-designed controlled trials using small samples, or guidelines developed from evidence and supported by expert opinion

CALENDULA

A large randomized controlled trial demonstrated the effectiveness of calendula compared to Biafine® (Ortho Dermatologics) for prevention of radiation-induced dermatitis. Pommier et al. (2004) randomized 254 women with breast cancer to using calendula or Biafine on irradiated fields after each treatment. Patients receiving calendula had less frequent interruptions of radiation therapy resulting from skin toxicity, lower prevalence of erythema, lower prevalence of grade 2 or higher acute dermatitis (p < 0.001), and lower levels of pain (p = 0.03) compared to the patients who used Biafine.

HYALURONIC ACID AND SODIUM HYALURONATE

A large double-blind, randomized, placebo-controlled trial demonstrated that the prophylactic use of hyaluronic acid cream (Ialugen®, Institut Biochimique) reduced the incidence of high-grade radiodermatitis. A case study also demonstrated the healing effect of hyaluronic acid. Expert opinion guidelines have recommended the use of hyaluronic acid topical cream in the management of grade 2 or 3 skin toxicity in the absence of infection (Bernier et al., 2008).

Liguori, Guillemin, Pesce, Mirimanoff, and Bernier (1997) randomly assigned 134 patients with head and neck, breast, or pelvic cancers to use of 0.2% hyaluronic acid cream or placebo. Subjects applied the topical cream once in the morning one to two hours after radiation therapy and once in the evening. Patients in the placebo group had higher severity of skin toxicity (p < 0.01). Global judgment of treatment efficacy was better with hyaluronic acid as judged by both patients (p < 0.05) and physicians (p < 0.01).

Bauer and Bauer (2009) published a single case report describing the effective use of topical sodium hyaluronate for severe radiation recall dermatitis, without discontinuation of the trigger drug. A woman with a complex history of multiple cancer treatments and chemotherapeutic regimens was given radiation therapy in preparation for an allogeneic bone marrow transplant. Three days after transplant she showed radiation recall dermatitis within the former radiation field. Treatment with topical sodium hyaluronate gel (Radiaplex™, MPH Medical) was administered twice daily, and marked improvement occurred within five days.

Benefits Balanced With Harms

Interventions for which clinicians and patients should weigh the beneficial and harmful effects according to individual circumstances and priorities

There are no interventions as of February 2010.

Effectiveness Not Established

Interventions for which insufficient or conflicting data or data of inadequate quality currently exist, with no clear indication of harm

A variety of topical and oral treatments, as well as various dressings, have been studied for their effects on radiation-induced skin toxicities. One systematic review examined results across 10 randomized controlled trials involving approximately 575 patients from 1990 to 2008 using various topical agents, hydrogel, or hydrocolloid dressings. It was concluded that no convincing evidence existed for any intervention studied (Kedge, 2009). Guidelines of the Cancer Care Ontario Supportive Care Guidelines Group also concluded that there was insufficient evidence to support or refute use of a variety of topical agents, IV agents, or oral agents (Bolderston et al., 2006).

TOPICAL AGENTS

Aloe Vera

Four individual research studies and a systematic review were found regarding the use of aloe vera. Vogler and Ernst (1999) looked at the results of 10 controlled clinical trials involving 740 subjects using aloe vera administered orally or as a topical agent. Both full published studies and study abstracts were included. Of these, two studies examined topical aloe vera for prevention or mitigation of radiodermatitis. The conclusion was that topical application does not seem to prevent radiation-induced skin damage and that it was not possible to draw firm conclusions from the review because of multiple research methodologic problems (Vogler & Ernst, 1999).

The four individual trials (Heggie et al., 2002; Merchant et al., 2007; Olsen et al., 2001; Williams et al., 1996) were all conducted as randomized controlled studies, and two were blinded. Two trials were conducted at multiple sites, and two were in single-site locations. Populations included patients receiving radiation for breast cancer and those with any radiated cancer site where skin reactions were expected to occur.

Merchant et al. (2007) compared aloe vera gel to an anionic polar phospholipid-based (APP) cream for prevention and treatment of radiation dermatitis in 45 pediatric patients receiving radiation therapy to the thorax, axilla, and craniocervical regions. Subjective assessment of skin comfort variables and CTC skin grades were analyzed. APP cream was found to be more effective than aloe vera gel for the prevention and treatment of radiodermatitis, and toxicity scores were lower in the APP group (p = 0.004).

Heggie et al. (2002) performed a double-blind, randomized controlled trial comparing topical aloe vera gel to the use of topical aqueous cream, a water-based moisturizing cream, in 208 females with breast cancer. Patients were stratified according to bra cup size, history of lymphocele drainage, and smoking. No overall differences were reported between the groups for pruritus, pain, erythema, or desquamation.

Olsen et al. (2001) compared the use of aloe and mild soap versus mild soap alone in 70 patients. Although the authors concluded that a protective effect of adding aloe to the care regimen seemed to occur, they did not provide actual data to support this conclusion. No significant differences were found between the study arms in skin texture, erythema, pruritus, tanning due to radiation therapy, or skin toxicity grades.

Williams et al. (1996) reported results of two randomized controlled trials. One trial compared aloe vera gel to a placebo gel, and the other compared aloe vera to no treatment. Both studies included females receiving radiation therapy for breast cancer as participants and included a total of 302 subjects. The first trial was double-blinded, used a placebo gel, and involved 194 women receiving breast or chest wall irradiation. The second trial randomized 108 such patients to aloe vera gel versus no treatment. No significant differences were observed between the groups in severity or prevalence of skin toxicities, and the authors concluded that results did not support a hypothesis that aloe vera could be used to decrease radiodermatitis (Williams et al., 1996).

Anionic Polar Phospholipid Cream
Merchant et al. (2007) tested the use of APP cream versus aloe vera gel in 45 pediatric patients with various cancers to determine effectiveness in preventing and treating radiation dermatitis. The two skin treatments were applied to adjacent areas of skin within the treatment field. Some patients and caregivers rated the APP cream as providing more comfort and less dryness than aloe vera. Overall results suggested that APP cream was more effective than the aloe vera gel by grouped common toxicity scores (p = 0.004); however, their sample size was small.

Bepanthen
Four clinical trials were found in which dexpanthenol (Bepanthen®, Bayer HealthCare) was compared to other treatments for the management of radiodermatitis (Løkkevik, Skovlund, Reitan, Hannisdal, & Tanum, 1996; Röper, Kaisig, Auer, Mergen, & Molls, 2004; Schmuth et al., 2002; Schreck, Pausen, Bamberg, & Budach, 2002). In three of these studies, Bepanthen was noted to be the institutional standard of care and was used as the study control arm. Only one study compared the use of Bepanthen to no topical treatment. All of these studies had very small sample sizes, and none were able to demonstrate an advantage with the use of Bepanthen.

Röper et al. (2004) compared the use of Bepanthen to theta cream in a randomized controlled study in 20 female patients with early-stage breast cancer. At an equivalent total dose of radiation, no differences were observed for maximal skin toxicity scores between groups.

Schreck et al. (2002) did a quasi-experimental design study in 12 patients with head and neck cancer by having patients apply different treatments to either side of the neck. They outlined a complex standard protocol for management of skin toxicities, which included the use of Bepanthen, and compared the use of cream and powder formulations in terms of skin toxicity and patient acceptance. Because of the small sample size, no statistical analysis was performed. Descriptive findings indicated no differences between treatments.

As summarized in the section under topical steroids, Schmuth et al. (2002) also tested the use of Bepanthen. This study showed no difference between those treated with Bepanthen and historical controls who were untreated.

Løkkevik et al. (1996) performed a quasi-experimental study in 79 patients with head and neck or breast cancer, testing Bepanthen against no topical treatment. Patients used Bepanthen on one side of the treatment field and no topical treatment on the other side of the field. No differences were seen in erythema, moist desquamation, pruritus, or pain. In this study, some patients were also receiving chemotherapy, but an analysis of this subgroup was not completed.

Chamomile Cream and Almond Ointment

Maiche, Gröhn, and Mäki-Hokkonen (1991) evaluated the use of Kamillosan® (AP Medical AB), an extract of the chamomile flower, versus the use of almond oil in 48 women receiving radiation for breast cancer. The patients served as their own controls, applying Kamillosan cream or almond oil to randomly determined sections of the radiation field prior to and after irradiation daily. Skin changes seemed to appear later in the Kamillosan group; however, a higher percentage of the Kamillosan group developed grade 3 reactions. Overall, no significant differences between the two groups were observed, and the conclusion was that neither of these topical treatments prevented skin reactions (Maiche et al., 1991).

Glutathione and Anthocyanin

One randomized, placebo-controlled trial evaluated the effectiveness of glutathione and anthocyanin (RayGel™, Integrative Therapies) among 30 females with breast cancer (Enomoto et al., 2005). Subjects were randomized to use RayGel versus a water-based gel that was dyed with beet juice to look like the RayGel. Skin toxicity was measured in terms of the total area of skin affected and worst skin score. Although some results appeared to be in favor of the RayGel, they were not statistically significant. Study findings were further compromised because all subjects were also instructed to use aloe vera and vitamin E.

Lipiderm

A prospective, randomized controlled trial examined the use of Lipiderm® (International Veterinary Sciences) versus Biafine for the prevention of radiation dermatitis in a sample of 74 patients receiving radiation for breast cancer. The study did not refute or support either product in terms of a protective effect (Fenig et al., 2001).

Sodium Sucrose Octasulfate

One study was found that tested the use of sodium sucrose octasulfate (NaSOS), a chemical somewhat similar to sucralfate, to prevent radiation-induced skin damage in patients with head and neck cancer (Evensen, Bjordal, Jacobsen, Løkkevik, & Tausjo, 2001). In this study, 60 patients served as their own controls applying NaSOS to one side of the neck and a placebo to the other side of the neck. The mean skin reaction values were somewhat higher with the use of the placebo (p = 0.012) (Evensen et al., 2001).

Steroids

Four randomized controlled trials were performed to examine the effectiveness of topical steroids for the prevention or management of radiodermatitis. All of these studies had small sample sizes and a number of methodologic issues in the research. None were able to demonstrate a clear benefit with the use of topical steroid treatments. Patients receiving chemotherapy were included in study samples, which can increase the potential for radiodermatitis. Furthermore, sample sizes were too small to allow for subgroup analysis.

Omidvari et al. (2007) compared betamethasone, petrolatum, and no treatment for acute radiation dermatitis prevention in 51 female patients who were undergoing radiation therapy for breast cancer. Skin toxicity initially increased for all groups, and the topical steroid use provided no clear benefit.

Shukla, Gairola, Mohanti, and Rath (2006) randomly assigned 60 patients who were undergoing radiation therapy for breast cancer to using beclomethasone spray or no intervention. The subjects who were using the beclomethasone had a lower prevalence of wet desquamation of the axilla than the control group (p = 0.037); however, they also reported no differences in the median dose of radiation that caused wet desquamation between groups. Thus, it was unclear if differences in prevalence of skin toxicity were associated with topical treatment or total radiation doses. All of these patients were treated on a telecobalt unit, which is generally associated with lower skin-sparing properties (Shukla et al., 2006).

Boström, Lindman, Swartling, Berne, and Bergh (2001) examined the use of mometasone furoate (MMF) in 50 females with breast cancer to determine if its use could reduce erythema intensity. Patients were randomized to use MMF or an emollient cream. The researchers calculated a total erythema score using spectrophotometry and reported a significantly lower maximal score among those treated with MMF (p = 0.011). Several methodologic issues were seen in this study, including that both groups used the placebo control cream, and compliance issues (Boström et al., 2001).

Schmuth et al. (2002) randomly assigned 23 women with breast cancer to use of either 0.1% methylprednisolone aceponate cream (Advantan®, Bayer HealthCare) or dexpanthenol (Bepanthen) and compared findings to those in an additional historical cohort of untreated patients. Patients treated with the steroid tended to have fewer high-grade skin reactions but were not better than the control group.

Sucralfate

Three studies were done to examine the effect of topical sucralfate for the prevention or management of radiodermatitis (Falkowski, Trouillas, Duroux, Bonnetblanc, & Clavère, 2009; Maiche, Isokangas, & Gröhn, 1994; Wells et al., 2004).

Falkowski et al. (2009) studied 21 female patients with breast cancer, using a quasi-experimental design. The skin zones in the radiation field were compared with one zone not in the radiation field. Spectrophotometry was used to measure skin responses, and skin toxicity was scored using the RTOG scale. No differences were reported between the areas treated with sucralfate and those not treated.

Wells et al. (2004) conducted a randomized, double-blind, controlled trial in 357 patients with head and neck, breast, or anorectal cancer. Subjects were randomized to one of six treatment combinations using an aqueous cream, sucralfate cream, or no cream. Within each group, subjects were randomized to either dry or hydrogel dressings. No differences were reported among the groups regarding time to moist desquamation, severity of skin reaction, or discomfort. Sucralfate cream was found to produce lower erythema readings with spectrophotometry than the aqueous cream, but the group treated with no cream had even lower readings.

Maiche et al. (1994) completed a quasi-experimental study with 44 female patients with breast cancer, in which participants applied sucralfate or a base cream to either side of their surgical scar. The side of the scar to receive the sucralfate was randomized, and researchers who graded the skin were blinded to treatment side. The study used a five-point scale that the researchers developed. No information regarding validity or reliability was discussed. Analysis of the patients who developed grade 1 or 2 skin reactions over the course of therapy showed that skin reactions tended to appear later on the skin treated with sucralfate, and at week 4 this difference was significant (p < 0.05). Recovery time of skin reaction was faster and the severity was lower with sucralfate (p = 0.05). They did not report whether any grade 3 or 4 skin reactions occurred.

Theta Cream
In one study, theta cream use was compared with Bepanthen use. This study, as previously described under Bepanthen, had a very small sample size. No differences were reported between the study groups, and neither topical treatment demonstrated any benefit (Röper et al., 2004).

Topical Vitamin C
Halperin, Gaspar, George, Darr, and Pinnell (1993) instructed 65 patients who were receiving radiation to the brain for metastatic disease to use a 10% ascorbic acid solution on one side of the radiation field and a vehicle control solution on the other side of the field. They found no benefit from use of the ascorbic acid lotion and no apparent differences in patient preference.

Urea Lotion
One study was found that investigated whether moist skin care with urea lotion (Eucerin®, Beiersdorf, Inc.) may reduce acute radiation skin toxicity. A study of 68 patients with head and neck cancer using moist skin care with 3% urea lotion was compared to dry skin care used in historical controls. Results showed that control subjects had a higher prevalence of skin toxicities at all grades, at lower doses of radiation, compared to patients using moist skin care with urea lotion ($p < 0.05$). The findings suggest that moist skin care with 3% urea lotion may delay acute radiodermatitis and grade 3 toxicities. However, many different factors, such as concomitant chemotherapy, variation in treatment field size, and type of radiation, were not considered in the analysis of the data and may have skewed the data (Momm, Weibenberger, Bartelt, & Henke, 2003).

XClair (MASO65D)
Two trials assessed the effect of XClair™ (Align Pharmaceuticals) in managing radiation dermatitis. Leonardi et al. (2008) randomly assigned 35 female subjects with breast cancer to topical treatment with XClair or a vehicle control. This study demonstrated less burning ($p = 0.039$) and desquamation ($p = 0.02$) and lower maximum skin toxicity grade ($p < 0.0001$) in the XClair group (Leonardi et al., 2008). Primavera et al. (2006) conducted a double-blind vehicle control with 22 female participants with breast cancer using XClair and the control topical agent to different sections of skin in the radiation field. No significant differences were observed between agents used for skin toxicity grades, erythema, pain, or pruritus (Primavera et al., 2006).

DRESSINGS

Nine studies were reviewed in which various skin dressings were used; four trials using hydrocolloid or hydrogel type dressings (Gollins, Gaffney, Slade, & Swindell, 2008; Macmillan et al., 2007; Mak, Molassiotis, Wan, Lee, & Chan, 2000; Mak et al., 2005), one using a no-sting barrier film (Cavilon™, 3M) (Graham et al., 2004), two studies using silver leaf dressings (Vavassis, Gelinas, Tr, & Nguyen-Tân, 2008; Vuong et al., 2004), one using honey-soaked gauze (Robson & Cooper, 2009), and one using granulocyte macrophage–colony-stimulating factor (GM-CSF) impregnated gauze (Kouvaris, Kouloulias, Plataniotis, Balafouta, & Vlahos, 2001). Kedge's 2009 systematic review also included studies of a variety of dressings.

Granulocyte Macrophage–Colony-Stimulating Factor

One study was done by Kouvaris et al. (2001) examining the effectiveness of GM-CSF impregnated gauze in preventing and healing acute radiodermatitis in 61 female patients with carcinoma of the vulva. Subjects all used steroid cream applications at the beginning of radiation therapy and used the GM-CSF gauze at the point they that received 20 Gy of radiation. Results in this group were compared to historical controls who had used betamethasone for prophylaxis throughout treatment. In this study, patients treated with GM-CSF had overall lower pain results ($p = 0.0014$) and less severe skin toxicity ($p = 0.008$) than historical controls. The study had a relatively small sample size as well as a lack of a prospective control group (Kouvaris et al., 2001).

Honey

Robson and Cooper (2009) reported a small case series of four patients who used honey as a primary dressing for managing radiation wounds with impaired healing. They reported in all cases that the change from conventional dressings to the topical application was followed by a noticeable improvement in healing.

Hydrocolloid Dressings

The evidence regarding the use of hydrogel and hydrocolloid dressings was mixed in a systematic review of randomized controlled studies. In some of the studies, patient comfort was seen with these interventions; however, some studies showed no differences. One study even showed increased healing time associated with the hydrogel dressing (Kedge, 2009).

Gollins et al. (2008) randomly assigned 30 patients with either head and neck cancer or breast cancer who had developed moist desquamation to the use of hydrogel dressing or gentian violet. The purpose was to determine differences in time to healing. The hydrogel group demonstrated a progressive reduction in the desquamation area. The median time to healing with hydrogel was 12 days compared to 30 days for gentian violet. The study was hampered by withdrawal of a large percentage of patients (62%) in the gentian violet group and the lack of a no-treatment arm for definitive comparisons.

Macmillan et al. (2007) also studied use of hydrogel in patients with moist desquamation The effect of a hydrogel versus nonadherent dressing in 100 patients with head and neck, anorectal, or breast cancer was reviewed. In this study, 357 patients were randomly assigned to treatment of desquamation at the beginning of radiation therapy and began to use the assigned treatment when moist desquamation occurred. The skin reactions of patients assigned to the hydrogel had a prolonged period of moist desquamation ($p = 0.03$). With the higher cost of the hydrogel and without supporting evidence of superior action, hydrogel was not recommended.

Mak et al. (2005) studied the use of nonadherent dressings in 142 patients who had unhealed wounds after irradiation. Patients were randomly assigned to use of the dressing or use of gentian violet. They found no significant differences between groups in wound healing, healing time, or other patient issues such as sleep, mood, and restriction of neck movement.

In another study, Mak et al. (2000) examined the use of hydrocolloid dressings for the management of moist desquamation. In this trial, 39 patients with various cancer diagnoses who had completed radiation therapy and had developed moist desquamation were randomly assigned to the use of gentian violet or hydrocolloid dressings. The analysis included consideration for whether concomitant chemotherapy was administered. No differences were found between the groups for healing time or pain.

No-Sting Barrier Film

Graham et al. (2004) studied the use of Cavilon no-sting barrier film versus glycerin cream in terms of skin toxicity and rates of moist desquamation in 58 females with breast cancer. Participants applied the control cream to one part of the irradiated field and the no-sting barrier to the alternate half of the field. If moist desquamation occurred, the treatment was switched over to the other treatment. This study found that no-sting barrier was associated with a lower total skin toxicity score (p = 0.0002) and a lower prevalence of pruritus (p = 0.017). The no-sting barrier was found to be more effective in reducing the duration and frequency of moist desquamation, but further studies are warranted (Graham et al., 2004).

Silver Leaf Dressings

Two studies were found that investigated the effectiveness of silver leaf dressings. One of these used silver leaf dressings to treat radiation-induced dermatitis, and one was conducted to evaluate their use in preventing radiodermatitis. Both of these were limited by very small sample sizes.

Vavassis et al. (2008) studied 12 patients with head and neck cancers who applied silver leaf dressings to one side of the neck and silver sulfadiazine to the other side of the neck for the treatment of radiodermatitis. No difference was reported in improvement of the skin reaction between the silver leaf dressing and the silver sulfadiazine control (Vavassis et al., 2008). However, the silver leaf dressing did reduce the severity of reaction within the same grade, accelerated healing, and provided improved pain control over silver sulfadiazine.

Vuong et al. (2004) compared 15 patients with anal or gynecologic cancers using silver leaf dressing versus historical controls using silver sulfadiazine at the occurrence of symptomatic dermatitis. All study patients used the silver leaf dressings starting day 1 of radiation until two weeks after treatment completion. Several observers from different institutions independently rated skin toxicity from digital photographs, and total mean scores across all observations were used in analysis. The mean dermatitis score among those using the silver leaf was significantly lower, leading to the authors' conclusion that the silver leaf dressing is effective in reducing radiation dermatitis (Vuoung et al., 2004). Some patients received concomitant chemotherapy and others did not, but because of the small sample, this factor was not considered in data analysis.

ORAL TREATMENTS

Oral agents studied for their effects on radiodermatitis include zinc (Lin, Que, Lin, & Lin, 2006), red wine (Morganti et al., 2009), sucralfate (Lievens et al.,1998), and proteolytic enzymes (Gujral et al., 2001).

Proteolytic Enzymes

Gujral et al. (2001) reported findings that using an oral proteolytic enzyme combination containing papain (100 mg), trypsin (40 mg) and chymotrypsin (40 mg) (Wobe-Mugos®, MU-COS Pharma) could prevent acute radiation side effects. The study was a prospective, randomized, open-label trial with 98 patients with head and neck cancer. Patients were given three tablets three times daily from three days prior to the start of radiation therapy until five days after the completion of therapy. Maximum skin toxicity was significantly lower in the enzyme-treated group (p < 0.00001). These findings suggest that further study in larger, more rigorously controlled studies would be beneficial (Gujral et al.).

Red Wine

Morganti et al. (2009) did a retrospective analysis of 348 females treated for breast cancer to evaluate the potential radioprotective effects of red wine. They found that the incidence of grade 2 or higher acute skin toxicity was higher in patients without red wine intake (p = 0.0021). Findings also varied according to the amount of daily red wine intake, with the best results seen in those who reported drinking one glass per day. No differences were observed between those with no alcohol intake and individuals who drank more or less than one glass per day.

Sucralfate

Lievens et al. (1998) did a randomized, placebo-controlled, double-blind study in 83 patients with head and neck cancer to see if oral sucralfate could reduce acute radiation-induced complications. The intervention was 1 gram of sucralfate ingested six times per day from the onset of radiotherapy until completion. They found no evidence that sucralfate reduced the acute side effects of radiation therapy.

Zinc

Lin et al. (2006) used zinc supplementation versus soybean oil placebo capsules in a randomized, double-blind, placebo-controlled study in 97 patients with head and neck cancer. Participants took 25 mg zinc or soybean oil placebo capsules three times per day. Grade 2 (p = 0.015) and grade 3 (p = 0.0092) dermatitis were less prevalent in those taking zinc across all weeks of therapy. Zinc also was found to delay the onset of dermatitis. Within the subset of patients who were also receiving chemotherapy, zinc supplementation did not show much benefit.

Effectiveness Unlikely

Interventions for which lack of effectiveness has been demonstrated by negative evidence from a single rigorously conducted controlled trial, consistent negative evidence from well-designed controlled trials using small samples, or guidelines developed from evidence and supported by expert opinion

TROLAMINE AND BIAFINE

Five studies (Elliott et al., 2006; Fenig et al., 2001; Fisher et al., 2000; Pommier et al., 2004; Szumacher et al., 2001) reported on the use of Biafine or trolamine for the prevention and management of radiodermatitis. The Pommier et al. (2004) study of 254 females treated for breast cancer was also discussed related to use of calendula. This study showed that patients treated with trolamine had worse results than those treated with calendula (Pommier et al., 2004).

Elliott et al. (2004) completed a multicenter phase III trial comparing a trolamine emulsion with best supportive care within each institution in 547 patients with head and neck cancer. Patients were randomly assigned to one of three treatment arms: (a) prophylactic trolamine, (b) use of trolamine as an intervention for dermatitis, or (c) the institutional best supportive care (1 of 14 products). The results demonstrated no advantage for the use of trolamine or differences across groups in the rates of grade 2 or higher radiodermatitis.

Fenig et al. (2001) conducted a randomized prospective trial at a single site with 74 patients with breast cancer who were receiving radiation. Patients were randomized to receive Biafine, Lipiderm, or no treatment. The results showed no advantage for either preparation compared to the no-treatment arm.

Szumacher et al. (2001) completed a phase II study of 60 patients with breast cancer that evaluated patients who had chemotherapy prior to radiation and the use of Biafine. Grade 2 radiation dermatitis was the most common, occurring in 85% of the study patients. These patients had no treatment delays or interruptions because of skin toxicity. No comparison groups were studied.

Fisher et al. (2000) conducted a multicenter trial with 172 analyzable patients with breast cancer. Biafine was compared to best supportive care at the institution or the no-treatment arm. In this study, patients were also stratified and data analyzed within groups by bra cup size. The study showed no difference in maximum skin toxicity or prevalence of grade 2 or higher skin toxicity between treatment arms. No differences were reported between Biafine and best supportive care in the prevention, time to, or duration of radiation-induced dermatitis. Biafine did seem to have a slight advantage in those with a larger bra cup size.

Not Recommended for Practice

Interventions for which lack of effectiveness or harmfulness has been demonstrated by strong evidence from rigorously conducted studies, meta-analyses, or systematic reviews, or interventions where the costs, burden, or harms associated with the intervention exceed anticipated benefit

GENTIAN VIOLET

Gentian violet has been described as a standard approach to care and has been used as the control treatment for the prevention or management of radiation-induced dermatitis in several studies (Gollins et al., 2008; Kedge, 2009; Mak et al., 2000, 2005). However, it is no longer recommended by the department of health in the United Kingdom because it has been shown to be carcinogenic in animals (Kedge, 2009). The tissue-damaging potency of the crystal violet dyes has been demonstrated in different experimental rat and rabbit models. The tissue-irritating effect of gentian violet has also given rise to controversy regarding its use on radiation-induced moist wounds (Eriksson & Mobacken, 1977; Mobacken, Zederfeldt, & Ahrén, 1973). In vitro, crystal violet was cytotoxic at low concentrations to HeLa cells and fibroblasts (Norrby & Mobacken, 1972). Although carcinogenicity of gentian violet is observed only in animals, its use has had some restrictions. For this reason, gentian violet is not recommended for practice.

Expert Opinion

Low-risk interventions that are (1) consistent with sound clinical practice, (2) suggested by an expert in a peer-reviewed publication (journal or book chapter), and (3) for which limited evidence exists. An expert is an individual with peer-reviewed journal publications in the domain of interest.

Personal Hygiene Habits and Recommendations for Care by Skin Toxicity Grade: Radiation Therapy and Epidermal Growth Factor Receptor Inhibitors

Consensus guidelines for patients receiving epidermal growth factor receptor inhibitors (Bernier et al., 2008) have presented skin care management guidance for the grade of dermatitis based on NCI criteria, and the Cancer Care Ontario Supportive Care Guidelines Group outlined many similar recommendations for care based upon its review of evidence (Bolderston et al., 2006). Considering these sources, general recommendations for care include

- Gentle skin washing with water or mild soap and water
- Gentle shampooing with mild shampoo if receiving radiation therapy to the head
- Encouragement of personal hygiene habits according to the patients' usual routine
- Avoidance of sun exposure and use of sun block or sunscreens with a sun protection factor of 15 or greater
- No use of straight razor on irradiated skin
- Establishing that skin reaction is not caused by other concomitant medications or patient conditions
- Individualized management according to the severity of skin toxicity in addition to general approaches as outlined.

Grade 1
- Can use optional moisturizer and anti-infective measures such as a triclosan- or chlorhexidine-based cream
- Management by the nurse

Grades 2 and 3
- Use topical approaches in the absence of infection.
- If infection is suspected, swab area to identify infectious agent. Topical antibiotic is not recommended.

Grade 4
- Wound care referral and management by wound specialists

General Recommendations

McQuestion (2006) identified and outlined various general recommendations for care based on clinical experience. General approaches for care include the following.
- Advise patients to wear loose clothing made from soft fabrics such as cotton.
- Avoid application of tape or adhesives to the treatment field.
- Advise patients to avoid use of cosmetic products such as perfume, makeup, and aftershave on skin in the treatment field.
- Do not use ice packs or heating pads on the skin in the treatment field.
- Instruct patients to avoid swimming in lakes or chlorinated pools or using hot tubs if skin had dry desquamation or more severe breakdown.

Areas for Research

The review of evidence suggests a number of important areas for research regarding the prevention and management of radiodermatitis. Current practice in this area demonstrates that a wide variety of treatments are used, and several randomized controlled studies have used comparison to standard practices that include interventions that do not have demonstrated effectiveness. This points to the need for greater attention to evidence-based practice in this area. The following are suggested areas for research.

- Studies need to be designed to address methodologic issues seen in current research.
  - Studies need to use comparison to true control groups or placebo controls rather than institutional standards or a multiplicity of other interventions. When studies attempt to compare outcomes across many different interventions, determining the effectiveness of any single approach or product is extremely difficult.
  - Research needs to be conducted with larger sample sizes. Many studies may show promising results; however, sample sizes tend to be inadequate to establish effectiveness.
  - Study end points need to be clear as to whether the goal is to prevent radiodermatitis, delay onset, facilitate healing, or reduce duration of dry or moist desquamation. Study designs need to enable analysis to answer relevant study questions.
  - The reliability and validity of skin grading and measurement tools used need to be determined and provided.
  - The timing of interventions and assessments in research needs to be clear and could benefit from more standardization. Timing and reporting according to radiation dose levels would be a more reproducible approach than timing according to number of days or weeks alone.
- More research in different patient populations is needed.
  - Little information is available for pediatric populations.
  - Although some of the studies that were reviewed included patients of various ethnicities, most of the studies had sample sizes that were too small to allow analysis of these groups separately. Research is needed that looks at the skin changes that occur with radiation in different ethnic populations.
  - Most studies were of patients with breast or head and neck cancers. Applicability of findings to other patient populations and radiation sites is not clear, and additional research is needed to address this.
- Improved skin grading scales and use of standard scales would be helpful. The fact that studies use many different approaches makes comparison across studies impossible. Commonly used scales, such as the RTOG, are not sensitive enough to pick up practical clinical differences. Research to identify more sensitive measures would be helpful.
- Intervention studies in patients receiving IMRT should be done. Most research has been done in groups receiving therapy with older technologies. As radiation treatment technology changes, study of interventions aimed at the prevention or management of skin toxicities needs to be conducted in concert with those changes.
- Silvadene, which is commonly used in clinical practice, has not been studied for its actual effectiveness in the radiation setting. This treatment, as well as others now used as institutional standards, should be studied.
- Studies should routinely include some common outcome measures, including assessment of pain, pruritus, patient distress, and patient preference or satisfaction.
- Further research regarding the potential effects of using deodorants containing aluminum needs to be done.

- Additional research with larger patient samples is warranted using those interventions that currently show the most promise. These include
  - Calendula
  - Hyaluronic acid
  - No-sting barrier
  - Silver leaf dressings.

Search Strategy

Computerized literature searching was done using the consolidated PICO terms as outlined below. An initial date range of 10 years was used, and additional manual retrieval was done for key findings from the literature. The limitations of adults and English language were used. The final literature search for evidence related to interventions was performed in February 2010.

Patient/Problem: Patients with cancer and skin reactions from radiation therapy or combined radiation therapy and chemotherapy or targeted therapy, hypopigmentation, hyperpigmentation, anhidrosis, ischemia, ulceration, necrosis, fibrosis, telangiectasia, dry desquamation, moist desquamation, radiation dermatitis, radiodermatitis, radiation recall, late effects, and scleroderma.

Intervention: Hyperbaric oxygen, GM-CSF impregnated gauze, amifostine, gentian violet, Aquaphor® (Beiersdorf, Inc.), Mepilex gel, sweeten cream, vitamin C, Radia-Guard® (Hope Medical Products, Inc.), Radiaplex® (MPM Medical, Inc.), ultraviolet light, photoprotection, cornstarch, pretreatment skin care, nutrition, complementary and alternative therapies, intensity modulated radiation therapy, washing, soap, deodorant, aluminum products, zinc, aloe vera, Biafine, trolamine, calendula, hyaluronic acid, corticosteroids/steroids, sucralfate, barrier film, DermaFilm® (DermaRite), Cavilon, no-sting barrier, sorbolene, antimicrobials, silver sulfadiazine, Silvadene® (Monarch Pharmaceuticals), silver dressings, Flamazine® (Smith & Nephew), hydrophilic ointments, gels, creams, lotions, hydrocolloid dressing, DuoDERM® (ConvaTec, Inc.), moisture vapor permeable dressings, mangosteen pericarp oil, mineral oil, Neosporin® (Johnson & Johnson), antibiotics, honey, red wine, olive oil, polyphenols, hydroxytyrosol, Hidrox® (CreAgri, Inc.), and Bepanthen

Comparison: Standard care, institutional preference, treatment modalities: intensity modulated radiation versus three-dimensional conformal

Outcomes: Radiation recall, wound healing, healing time, duration of radiation dermatitis, onset of radiation dermatitis, pain, quality of life, reduced severity, long-term effects, fungal infection, bacterial infection, surgical wound healing

Type of Intervention: Prevention, treatment, management

Databases Used: PubMed, CINAHL®, EMBASE®, Cochrane Collaboration

Limits: Humans, English language

Definitions of the interventions are available at **www.ons.org/research/PEP**. Literature search completed through February 2010.

References

Bauer, S.M., & Bauer, C. (2009). The use of sodium hyaluronate for the treatment of radiation recall dermatitis. *Journal of Oncology Pharmacy Practice, 15,* 123–126. doi:10.1177/1078155208099705

Bernier, J., Bonner, J., Vermorken, J.B., Bensadoun, R.-J., Dummer, R., Giralt, J., ... Ang, K.K. (2008). Consensus guidelines for the management of radiation dermatitis and coexisting acne-like rash in patients receiving radiotherapy plus EGFR inhibitors for the treatment of squamous cell carcinoma of the head and neck. *Annals of Oncology, 19,* 142–149. doi:10.1093/annonc/mdm400

Bolderston, A., Lloyd, N.S., Wong, R.K.S., Holden, L., Robb-Blenderman, L., & Supportive Care Guidelines Group. (2006). *The prevention and management of acute skin reactions related to radiation therapy: A clinical practice guideline* (Practice Guidelines Report #13-7). Toronto, Ontario, Canada: Cancer Care Ontario.

Boström, A., Lindman, H., Swartling, C., Berne, B., & Bergh, J. (2001). Potent corticosteroid cream (mometasone furoate) significantly reduces acute radiation dermatitis: Results from a double-blind, randomized study. *Radiotherapy and Oncology, 59,* 257–265. doi:10.1016/S0167-8140(01)00327-9

Burch, S.E., Parker, S.A., Vann, A.M., & Arazie, J.C. (1997). Measurement of 6-MV x-ray surface dose when topical agents are applied prior to external beam irradiation. *International Journal of Radiation Oncology, Biology, Physics, 38,* 447–451. doi:10.1016/S0360-3016(97)00095-3

Campbell, I.R., & Illingworth, M.H. (1992). Can patients wash during radiotherapy to the breast or chest wall? A randomized controlled trial. *Clinical Oncology, 4,* 78–82.

Elliott, E.A., Wright, J.R., Swann, R.S., Nguyen-Tân, F., Takita, C., Bucci, M.K., ... Berk, L. (2006). Phase III trial of an emulsion containing trolamine for the prevention of radiation dermatitis in patients with advanced squamous cell carcinoma of the head and neck: Results of Radiation Therapy Oncology Group Trial 99-13. *Journal of Clinical Oncology, 24,* 2092–2096. doi:10.1200/JCO.2005.04.9148

Enomoto, T.M., Johnson, T., Peterson, N., Homer, L., Walts, D., & Johnson, N. (2005). Combination glutathione and anthocyanins as an alternative for skin care during external-beam radiation. *American Journal of Surgery, 189,* 627–631. doi:10.1016/j.amjsurg.2005.02.001

Eriksson, E., & Mobacken, H. (1977). Microvascular effects of a topically applied cationic triphenylmethane dye (crystal violet). *Acta Dermato-Venereologica, 57,* 45–49.

Evensen, J.F., Bjordal, K., Jacobsen, A.-B., Løkkevik, E., & Tausjø, J.E. (2001). Effects of Na-sucrose octasulfate on skin and mucosa reactions during radiotherapy of head and neck cancers. *Acta Oncologica, 40,* 751–755.

Falkowski, S., Trouillas, P., Duroux, J.-L., Bonnetblanc, J.-M., & Clavère, P. (2009). Radiodermatitis prevention with sucralfate in breast cancer: Fundamental and clinical studies. Advance online publication. *Supportive Care in Cancer.* doi:10.1007/s00520-009-0788-y

Fenig, E., Brenner, B., Katz, A., Sulkes, J., Lapidot, M., Schachter, J., ... Gutman, H. (2001). Topical Biafine and Lipiderm for the prevention of radiation dermatitis: A randomized prospective trial. *Oncology Reports, 8,* 305–309.

Fisher, J., Scott, C., Stevens, R., Marconi, B., Champion, L., Freedman, G.M., ... Wong, G. (2000). Randomized phase III study comparing best supportive care to Biafine as a prophylactic agent for radiation-induced skin toxicity for women undergoing breast irradiation: Radiation Therapy Oncology Group (RTOG) 97-13. *International Journal of Radiation Oncology, Biology, Physics, 48,* 1307–1310. doi:10.1016/S0360-3016(00)00782-3

Freedman, G.M., Anderson, P.R., Li, J., Jinsheng, L., Eisenberg, D.F., Hanlon, A.L., ... Nicolaou, N. (2006). Intensity modulated radiation therapy (IMRT) decreases acute skin toxicity for women receiving radiation for breast cancer. *American Journal of Clinical Oncology, 29,* 66–70. doi:10.1097/01.coc.0000197661.09628.03

Freedman, G.M., Li, T., Nicolaou, N., Chen, Y., Ma, C.C.-M., & Anderson, P.R. (2009). Breast intensity-modulated radiation therapy reduces time spent with acute dermatitis for women of all breast sizes during radiation. *International Journal of Radiation Oncology, Biology, Physics, 74,* 689–694. doi:10.1016/j.ijrobp.2008.08.071

Gollins, S., Gaffney, C., Slade, S., & Swindell, R. (2008). RCT on gentian violet versus a hydrogel dressing for radiotherapy-induced moist skin desquamation. *Journal of Wound Care, 17,* 268–275.

Graham, P., Browne, L., Capp, A., Fox, C., Graham, J., Hollis, J., & Nasser, E. (2004). Randomized, paired comparison of no-sting barrier film versus sorbolene cream (10% glycerine) skin care during post mastectomy irradiation. *International Journal of Radiation Oncology, Biology, Physics, 58,* 241–246. doi:10.1016/S0360-3016(03)01431-7

Gujral, M.S., Patnaik, P.M., Kaul, R., Parikh, H.K., Conradt, C., Tamhankar, C.P., & Daftary, G.V. (2001). Efficacy of hydrolytic enzymes in preventing radiation therapy-induced side effects in patients with head and neck cancers. *Cancer Chemotherapy and Pharmacology, 47*(Suppl.), S23–S28. doi:10.1007/s002800170005

Halperin, E.D., Gaspar, L., George, S., Darr, D., & Pinnell, S. (1993). A double-blind, randomized, prospective trial to evaluate topical vitamin C solution for the prevention of radiation dermatitis. *International Journal of Radiation Oncology, Biology, Physics, 26,* 413–416.

Heggie, S., Bryant, G.P., Tripcony, L., Keller, J., Rose, P., Glendenning, M., & Heath, J. (2002). A phase III study on the efficacy of topical aloe vera gel on irradiated breast tissue. *Cancer Nursing, 25,* 442–451.

Kedge, E.M. (2009). A systematic review to investigate the effectiveness and acceptability of interventions for moist desquamation in radiotherapy patients. *Radiography, 15,* 247–257. doi:10.1016/j.radi.2008.08.002

Kouvaris, J.R., Kouloulias, V.E., Plataniotis, G.A., Balafouta, E.J., & Vlahos, L.J. (2001). Dermatitis during radiation for vulvar carcinoma: Prevention and treatment with granulocyte-macrophage colony-stimulating factor impregnated gauze. *Wound Repair and Regeneration, 9,* 187–193.

Leonardi, M.C., Gariboldi, S., Ivaldi, G.B., Ferrari, A., Serafini, F., Didier, F., … Orecchia, R. (2008). A double-blind, randomised, vehicle-controlled clinical study to evaluate the efficacy of MAS065D in limiting the effects of radiation on the skin: Interim analysis. *European Journal of Dermatology, 18,* 317–321. doi:10.1684/ejd.2008.0396

Lievens, Y., Haustermans, K., Van den Weyngaert, D., Van den Bogaert, W., Scalliet, P., Hutsebaut, L., … Lambin, P. (1998). Does sucralfate reduce the acute side-effects in head and neck cancer treated with radiotherapy? A double-blind randomized trial. *Radiotherapy and Oncology, 47,* 149–153.

Liguori, V., Guillemin, C., Pesce, G.F., Mirimanoff, R.O., & Bernier, J. (1997). Double-blind, randomized clinical study comparing hyaluronic acid cream to placebo in patients treated with radiotherapy. *Radiotherapy and Oncology, 42,* 155–161. doi:10.1016/S0167-8140(96)01882-8

Lin, L.-C., Que, J., Lin, L.-K., & Lin, F.-C. (2006). Zinc supplementation to improve mucositis and dermatitis in patients after radiotherapy for head-and-neck cancers: A double-blind, randomized study. *International Journal of Radiation Oncology, Biology, Physics, 65,* 745–750. doi:10.1016/j.ijrobp.2006.01.015

Løkkevik, E., Skovlund, E., Reitan, J.B., Hannisdal, E., & Tanum, G. (1996). Skin treatment with Bepanthen cream versus no cream during radiotherapy. *Acta Oncologica, 35,* 1021–1026.

Macmillan, M.S., Wells, M., MacBride, S., Raab, G.M., Munro, A., & MacDougall, H. (2007). Randomized comparison of dry dressings versus hydrogel in management of radiation-induced moist desquamation. *International Journal of Radiation Oncology, Biology, Physics, 68,* 864–872. doi:10.1016/j.ijrobp.2006.12.049

Maiche, A., Isokangas, O.-P., & Gröhn, P. (1994). Skin protection by sucralfate cream during electron beam therapy. *Acta Oncologica, 33,* 201–203.

Maiche, A.G., Gröhn, P., & Mäki-Hokkonen, H. (1991). Effect of chamomile cream and almond ointment on acute radiation skin reaction. *Acta Oncologica, 30,* 395–396.

Mak, S.S., Molassiotis, A., Wan, W.-M., Lee, I.Y.M., & Chan, E.S.J. (2000). The effects of hydrocolloid dressing and gentian violet on radiation-induced moist desquamation wound healing. *Cancer Nursing, 23,* 220–229.

Mak, S.S., Zee, C.Y., Molassiotis, A., Chan, S.J., Leung, S.F., Mo, K.F., & Johnson, P.J. (2005). A comparison of wound treatments in nasopharyngeal cancer patients receiving radiation therapy. *Cancer Nursing, 28,* 436–445.

McQuestion, M. (2006). Evidence-based skin care management in radiation therapy. *Seminars in Oncology Nursing, 27,* 163–173. doi:10.1016/j.soncn.2006.04.004

McQuestion, M. (2010). Radiation-induced skin reactions. In M.L. Haas & G.J. Moore-Higgs (Eds.), *Principles of skin care and the oncology patient* (pp. 115–140). Pittsburgh, PA: Oncology Nursing Society.

Meegan, M.A., & Haycocks, T.R. (1997). An investigation into the management of acute skin reactions from tangential breast irradiation. *Canadian Journal of Medical Radiation, 28,* 169–173.

Merchant, T.E., Bosley, C., Smith, J., Baratti, P., Pritchard, D., Davis, T., … Xiong, X. (2007). A phase III trial comparing an anionic phospholipid-based cream and aloe vera-based gel in the prevention of radiation dermatitis in pediatric patients. *Radiation Oncology, 2,* 45. doi:10.1186/1748-717X-2-45

Mobacken, H., Zederfeldt, B., & Ahrén, C. (1973). Effects of two cationic triphenylmethane dyes on the healing of skin incisions: A tensiometric and histologic study in the rat. *Acta Dermato-Venereologica, 53,* 161–166.

Momm, F., Weibenberger, C., Bartelt, S., & Henke, M. (2003). Moist skin care can diminish acute radiation-induced skin toxicity. *Strahlentherapie und Onkologie, 179,* 708–712. doi:10.1007/s00066-003-1142-9

Morganti, A.G., Digesù, C., Panunzi, S., de Gaetano, A., Macchia, G., Deodato, F., … de Gaetano, G. (2009). Radioprotective effect of moderate wine consumption in patients with breast carcinoma. *International Journal of Radiation Oncology, Biology, Physics, 74,* 1501–1505. doi:10.1016/j.ijrobp.2008.10.089

Norrby, K., & Mobacken, H. (1972). Effect of triphenylmethane dyes (brilliant green, crystal violet, methyl violet) on proliferation in human normal fibroblast-like and established epithelial-like cell lines. *Acta Dermato-Venereologica, 52,* 476–483.

Olsen, D.L., Raub, W., Jr., Bradley, C., Johnson, M., Macias, J.L., Love, V., & Markoe, A. (2001). The effect of aloe vera gel/mild soap versus mild soap alone in preventing skin reactions in patients undergoing radiation therapy. *Oncology Nursing Forum, 28,* 543–547.

Omidvari, S., Saboori, H., Mohammadianpanah, M., Mosalaei, A., Ahmadloo, N., Mosleh-Shirazi, M.A., … Namaz, S. (2007). Topical betamethasone for prevention of radiation dermatitis. *Indian Journal of Dermatology, Venereology and Leprology, 73,* 209–214.

Pignol, J.P., Olivotto, I., Rakovitch, E., Gardner, S., Sixel, K., Beckham, W., … Paszat, L. (2008). A multi-center randomized trial of breast intensity-modulated radiation therapy to reduce acute radiation dermatitis. *Journal of Clinical Oncology, 26,* 2085–2092. doi:10.1200/JCO.2007.15.2488

Pommier, P., Gomez, F., Sunyach, M.P., D'Hombres, A., Carrie, C., & Montbarbon, X. (2004). Phase III randomized trial of calendula officinalis compared with trolamine for the prevention of acute dermatitis during irradiation for breast cancer. *Journal of Clinical Oncology, 22,* 1447–1453. doi:10.1200/JCO.2004.07.063

Primavera, G., Carrera, M., Berardesca, E., Pinnaró, P., Messina, M., & Arcangeli, G. (2006). A double-blind, vehicle-controlled clinical study to evaluate the efficacy of MAS065D (XClair), a hyaluronic acid-based formulation, in the management of radiation-induced dermatitis. *Cutaneous and Ocular Toxicology, 25,* 165–171. doi:10.1080/15569520600860009

Robson, V., & Cooper, R. (2009). Using leptospermum honey to manage wounds impaired by radiotherapy: A case series. *Ostomy/Wound Management, 55,* 38–47.

Röper, B., Kaisig, D., Auer, F., Mergen, E., & Molls, M. (2004). Theta-cream versus bepanthol lotion in breast cancer patients under radiotherapy. *Strahlentherapie und Onkologie, 180,* 315–322. doi:10.1007/s00066-004-1174-9

Roy, I., Fortin, A., & Larochelle, M. (2001). The impact of skin washing with water and soap during breast irradiation: A randomized study. *Radiotherapy and Oncology, 58,* 333–339.

Schmuth, M., Wimmer, M.A., Hofer, S., Sztankay, A., Weinlich, G., Linder, D.M., … Fritsch, E. (2002). Topical corticosteroid therapy for acute radiation dermatitis: A prospective, randomized, double-blind study. *British Journal of Dermatology, 146,* 983–991. doi:10.1046/j.1365-2133.2002.04751.x

Schreck, U., Pausen, F., Bamberg, M., & Budach, W. (2002). Intraindividual comparison of two different skin care conceptions in patients undergoing radiotherapy of the head-and-neck region: Creme or powder? *Strahlentherapie und Onkologie, 178,* 321–329.

Shukla, P.N., Gairola, M., Mohanti, B.K., & Rath, G.K. (2006). Prophylactic beclomethasone spray to the skin during postoperative radiotherapy of carcinoma breast: A prospective randomized study. *Indian Journal of Cancer, 43,* 180–184. doi:10.4103/0019-509X.29424

Szumacher, E., Wighton, A., Franssen, E., Chow, E., Tsao, M., Ackerman, I., … Hayter, C. (2001). Phase II study assessing the effectiveness of Biafine cream as a prophylactic agent for radiation-induced acute skin toxicity to the breast in women undergoing radiotherapy with concomitant CMF chemotherapy. *International Journal of Radiation Oncology, Biology, Physics, 51,* 81–86. doi:10.1016/S0360-3016(01)01576-0

Théberge, V., Harel, F., & Dagnault, A. (2009). Use of axillary deodorant and effect on acute skin toxicity during radiotherapy for breast cancer: A prospective randomized noninferiority trial. *International Journal of Radiation Oncology, Biology, Physics, 75,* 1048–1052. doi:10.1016/j.ijrobp.2008.12.046

Vavassis, P., Gelinas, M., Tr, J.C., & Nguyen-Tân, P.F. (2008). Phase 2 study of silver leaf dressing for treatment of radiation-induced dermatitis in patients receiving radiotherapy to the head and neck. *Journal of Otolaryngology-Head and Neck Surgery, 37,* 124–129.

Vogler, B.K., & Ernst, E. (1999). Aloe vera: A systematic review of its clinical effectiveness. *British Journal of General Practice, 49,* 823–828. Retrieved from http://www.ncbi.nlm.nih.gov/pmc/articles/PMC1313538/?tool=pubmed

Vuong, R., Franco, E., Lehnert, S., Lambert, C., Portelance, L., Nasr, E., … Freeman, C. (2004). Silver leaf nylon dressing to prevent radiation dermatitis in patients undergoing chemotherapy and external beam radiotherapy to the perineum. *International Journal of Radiation Oncology, Biology, Physics, 59,* 809–814. doi:10.1016/j.ijrobp.2003.11.031

Wells, M., Macmillan, M., Raab, G., MacBride, S., Bell, N., MacKinnon, K., … Munro, A. (2004). Does aqueous or sucralfate cream affect the severity of erythematous radiation skin reactions? A randomized controlled trial. *Radiotherapy and Oncology, 73,* 153–162. doi:10.1016/j.ijrobp.2003.11.031

Westbury, C., Hines, F., Hawkes, E., Ashley, S., & Brada, M. (2000). Advice on hair and scalp care during cranial radiotherapy: A prospective randomized trial. *Radiotherapy and Oncology, 54,* 109–116. doi:10.1016/S0167-8140(99)00146-2

Williams, M.S., Burk, M., Loprinzi, C.L., Hill, M., Schomberg, P.J., Nearhood, K., ... Eggleston, W.D. (1996). Phase III double-blind evaluation of an aloe vera gel as a prophylactic agent for radiation-induced skin toxicity. *International Journal of Radiation Oncology, Biology, Physics, 36,* 345–349. doi:10.1016/S0360 -3016(96)00320-3

CHAPTER 5

Skin Reactions:
Rash, Palmar-Plantar Erythrodysesthesia, Xerosis, Paronychia, Photosensitivity, and Pruritus

Editor, Jeanene (Gigi) Robison, MSN, RN, AOCN®

Problem

Cutaneous reactions to chemotherapy and biotherapy can be mild, moderate, or severe. Although these reactions are rarely life threatening, they can significantly affect patients' quality of life, physical abilities, and psychosocial well-being (Burtness et al., 2009; de Noronha e Menezes et al., 2009; Lynch et al., 2007).

A variety of potential skin reactions related to cancer treatment can affect the patient's skin, hair, and nails. This chapter will be limited to the following skin reactions, which are those that are most often encountered and have interventions that have been reported: rash, palmar-plantar erythrodysesthesia (PPE), xerosis, paronychia, photosensitivity, and pruritus.

The two major types of rashes seen are acneform and maculopapular rash. Acneform rash generally presents as a diffuse erythema over the face and body, progressing to follicular papules and pustules resembling acne (National Cancer Institute Cancer Therapy Evaluation Program [NCI CTEP], 2010; Polovich, Whitford, & Olsen, 2009). Maculopapular rash is characterized by the presence of flat macules and elevated papules. This type of rash frequently affects the upper trunk, spreads centripetally, and is associated with pruritus (NCI CTEP, 2010).

The clinical manifestations of skin rash have many variables because of the unique differences in the agents used and their mechanism of action (Esper, Gale, & Muehlbauer, 2007). For example, carboplatin may cause allergic reactions, which can manifest as dermatologic reactions, including a rash, urticaria, erythema, and pruritus (Wilkes & Barton-Burke, 2010). Skin reactions caused by interleukin-2 may include an erythematous rash, pruritus, and dry and peeling skin (Schwartzentruber, 2000). Patients treated with interferon alfa have experienced more diffuse skin reactions that may be caused by immunologic and inflammatory mechanisms (Esper et al., 2007). The pathophysiology of the rash associated with epidermal growth factor receptor (EGFR) inhibitor therapy is not completely understood, but this therapy is believed to be related to the role of the EGFR in protecting and maintaining the integrity of the skin. When EGFR is inhibited, disruption in the growth and differentiation creates characteristic dermatologic effects (Eaby, Culkin, & Lacouture, 2008; Viale, 2010).

PPE (also known as hand-foot syndrome) first appears as mild redness and discomfort on the palms and soles with tingling sensations in the hands, usually at the fingertips. Symptoms progress to a more intense burning pain and tenderness, swelling, desquamation, severe crusting, ulceration, and epidermal necrosis (NCI CTEP, 2010; Polovich et al., 2009; Rossi et al., 2007).

Xerosis is characterized by abnormally dry, flaky, and dull skin (NCI CTEP, 2010; Polovich et al., 2009). Paronychia is painful inflammation of tissue around fingernails and toenails, more commonly seen in great toes and thumbs (Polovich et al., 2009). Photosensitivity appears as an erythematous response to ultraviolet or visible light (Dubakiene & Kupriene, 2006; NCI CTEP, 2010; Polovich et al., 2009). Pruritus is intense itching that may lead to scratching and is often associated with rash and xerosis (Dest, 2010; NCI CTEP, 2010; Polovich et al., 2009).

An overview of interventions that have been studied for the skin reactions discussed in this chapter and the resource is shown in Table 5-1.

Incidence

Multiple chemotherapy and biotherapy drugs can cause various skin reactions, and the incidence of specific skin toxicities varies with the treatment drugs used. With the advancement in the treatment of patients with targeted therapies, such as EGFR inhibitors, the incidence of skin reactions has increased (Lacouture, Basti, Patel, & Benson, 2006). Two classes of EGFR inhibitors are associated with skin reactions: monoclonal antibodies (MoAbs) and tyrosine kinase inhibitors (TKIs). The skin toxicities associated with different chemotherapy and biotherapy drugs are shown in Table 5-2.

Rash

The most common dermatologic adverse event is skin rash. The incidence of rash varies for different drugs. For patients receiving MoAbs, rash occurs in up to 80%–90% of patients receiving cetuximab therapy and in 90%–100% of patients receiving the maximum dose of panitumumab (Lacouture et al., 2006; Melosky et al., 2009; Molinari, De Quatrebarbes, André, & Aractingi, 2005; Scope et al., 2007; Segaert & Van Cutsem, 2005).

For patients who receive TKIs, rash occurs in 37%–65% of patients receiving gefitinib therapy and 67%–79% of patients receiving erlotinib therapy. The rash develops one to three weeks after therapy initiation, and the severity of the rash tends to be worse with the MoAbs (Bianchini, Jayanth, Chua, & Cunningham, 2008; Esper

Table 5-1. Intervention Evidence and Application to Skin Toxicity Type

Intervention Type	Skin Toxicity Type	Comments
Local and Regional Interventions		
Combined acetic acid soaks, salicylic acid, topical agents and systemic antibiotics	Rash	One case report
Regional cooling	PPE	Studies and case report show mixed results.
Topical Agent Interventions		
Antibiotics	Rash, paronychia	Six reports and case studies with EGFR inhibitor rash or paronychia and one systematic review In most cases, topical antibiotics combined with other interventions or discontinuation of cancer treatment
Bag Balm®, Dairy Association, Inc.	PPE	One study in patients receiving various chemotherapy agents
Benzoyl peroxide	Rash	Case reports with EGFR inhibitor rash combined with topical retinoid NCCN suggests not indicated for EGFR inhibitor rash
DMSO	PPE	One report of two patients receiving PLD
Elidel®, Novartis Pharmaceuticals (immune modulator)	Rash, pruritus	One case report with EGFR inhibitor therapy; combined with systemic antibiotics
Moisturizers and emollients	Rash, pruritus, PPE, xerosis	Five studies, four case series, three case reports Topical agents often combined with other topical treatment, systemic antibiotics, or holding cancer treatment
Retinoids	Rash, photosensitivity	Two studies, two case series, one case study EGFR inhibitor and other chemotherapies Combined with systemic retinoids, topical steroids, and topical antiseptics
Steroids	Rash, photosensitivity	One case study, systematic review, and NCCN Task Force Report
Systemic Interventions and Medications		
Amifostine	PPE	Used in two cancer treatment studies

(Continued on next page)

Table 5-1. Intervention Evidence and Application to Skin Toxicity Type
(Continued)

Intervention Type	Skin Toxicity Type	Comments
Systemic Interventions and Medications *(Cont.)*		
Antibiotics	Rash, xerosis, pruritus, paronychia	Three studies, one systematic review, multiple case series and reports, most in EGFR inhibitor therapy Case reports note combined interventions, including withholding cancer therapy
COX-2 inhibitors	Paronychia	One retrospective study
Pregabalin	Rash, PPE	One case report
Pyridoxine	PPE	Seven case studies, one retrospective study Used in combination with multiple interventions
Vitamin E	Paronychia	One case study
Other Interventions		
Electrodessication	Paronychia	One case study
Minimizing sun exposure	Photosensitivity	Two case studies with EGFR inhibitor therapy
Nicotine patch	PPE	One case report

COX-2—cyclooxygenase-2; DMSO—dimethyl sulfoxide; EGFR—epidermal growth factor receptor; NCCN—National Comprehensive Cancer Network; PLD—pegylated liposomal doxorubicin; PPE—palmar-plantar erythrodysesthesia

et al., 2007; Herbst, LoRusso, Purdom, & Ward, 2003; Jia, Lacouture, Su, & Wu, 2009; Micantonio et al., 2005; Oishi, 2008; Scope et al., 2007).

Rash occurs in 50%–100% of patients receiving chemotherapy regimens with high-dose cytarabine for induction or consolidation of acute myeloid leukemia (Wright, 2006).

Palmar-Plantar Erythrodysesthesia

PPE can be a dose-limiting toxicity for several chemotherapy agents, including capecitabine, continuous infusion fluorouracil (5-FU), pegylated liposomal doxorubicin (PLD or Doxil® [Ortho Biotech Products]), and docetaxel. The incidence of PPE has been found to be dose and schedule dependent (Drake et al., 2004). For patients receiving capecitabine, the overall incidence of PPE is 45%–65% (Heo et al., 2004). The incidence of PPE is associated with capecitabine dose, with 76% of patients experiencing PPE in the highest dose ranges, compared

Table 5-2. Chemotherapy and Biotherapy Drugs and Associated Risk for Developing Selected Skin Toxicities

Treatment Type	Xerosis	Paronychia	Photosensitivity	PPE	Pruritus	Rash
Chemotherapy						
Altretamine (Hexalen®, U.S. Bioscience)					X	X
Arsenic trioxide (Trisenox®, Cephalon Oncology)	X				X	X
Bleomycin (Blenoxane®, Bristol-Myers Squibb)		X	X		X	X
Busulfan (Busulfex®, Otsuka America Pharmaceutical)					X	X
Capecitabine (Xeloda®, Genentech)	X			X	X	
Carboplatin (Paraplatin®, Bristol-Myers Squibb)					X	X
Cisplatin (Platinol®, Bristol-Myers Squibb)					X	
Cladribine (Leustatin®, Ortho Biotech; 2-CdA)					X	X
Cyclophosphamide (Cytoxan®, Bristol-Myers Squibb)		X			X	
Cytarabine (ARA-C)				X	X	X
Dacarbazine (DTIC-Dome®, Bayer Pharmaceuticals)			X		X	X
Dactinomycin (actinomycin, Cosmegen®, Ovation Pharmaceuticals)			X		X	X
Daunorubicin (Daunomycin®, Bedford Laboratories)					X	X
Docetaxel (Taxotere®, sanofi-aventis)		X		X	X	X
Doxorubicin (Adriamycin®, Bedford Laboratories)		X	X	X	X	X
Doxorubicin, pegylated liposomal (PLD; Doxil®, Ortho Biotech)			X	X	X	X
Etoposide (VP-16)					X	

(Continued on next page)

Table 5-2. Chemotherapy and Biotherapy Drugs and Associated Risk for Developing Selected Skin Toxicities (Continued)

Treatment Type	Xerosis	Paronychia	Photosensitivity	PPE	Pruritus	Rash
Chemotherapy (Cont.)						
Floxuridine (FUDR®, Mayne Pharma)			X	X	X	X
Fludarabine (Fludara®, Bayer HealthCare Pharmaceuticals)					X	X
Fluorouracil (5-FU; Adrucil®, Teva Parenteral Medicines)	X		X	X (continuous infusion)	X	
Gemcitabine (Gemzar®, Eli Lilly)			X		X	X
Hydroxyurea (Hydrea®, Bristol-Myers Squibb)		X	X		X	X
Idarubicin (Idamycin®, Pharmacia and Upjohn)			X	X	X	X
Melphalan (Alkeran®, GlaxoSmithKline)					X	X
Methotrexate (MTX)		X	X		X	X (high dose)
Pemetrexed (Alimta®, Eli Lilly)					X	X
Pentostatin (Nipent®, Hospira)					X	X
Temozolomide (Temodar®, Schering Corp.)			X		X	X
Thiotepa (Thioplex®, Amgen)					X	X
Vinblastine (Velban®, Eli Lilly)			X		X	X

(Continued on next page)

Table 5-2. Chemotherapy and Biotherapy Drugs and Associated Risk for Developing Selected Skin Toxicities *(Continued)*

Treatment Type	Xerosis	Paronychia	Photosensitivity	PPE	Pruritus	Rash
Biotherapy: Monoclonal Antibodies						
Alemtuzumab (Campath®, Bayer HealthCare Pharmaceuticals)						X
Cetuximab (Erbitux®, Eli Lilly/Bristol-Myers Squibb)	X	X	X		X	X
Gemtuzumab ozogamicin (Mylotarg®, Wyeth Pharmaceuticals)						X
Ibritumomab tiuxetan (Zevalin®, Spectrum Pharmaceuticals)						X
Panitumumab (Vectibix®, Amgen)	X	X	X		X	X
Rituximab (Rituxan®, Genentech)						X
Tositumomab I-131 (Bexxar®, GlaxoSmithKline)	X					X
Trastuzumab (Herceptin®, Genentech)						X
Biotherapy: Small Molecule Inhibitors						
Erlotinib (Tarceva®, OSI Pharmaceuticals)	X				X	X
Gefitinib (Iressa®, AstraZeneca Pharmaceuticals)	X				X	X
Imatinib mesylate (Gleevec®, Novartis Pharmaceuticals)					X	X
Lapatinib (Tykerb®, GlaxoSmithKline)	X			X		X
Nilotinib (Tasigna®, Novartis Pharmaceuticals)					X	X
Sorafenib (Nexavar®, Bayer HealthCare Pharmaceuticals)	X			X	X	X
Sunitinib (Sutent®, Pfizer)	X			X		X
Temsirolimus (Torisel®, Wyeth Pharmaceuticals)	X				X	X

(Continued on next page)

Table 5-2. Chemotherapy and Biotherapy Drugs and Associated Risk for Developing Selected Skin Toxicities *(Continued)*

Treatment Type	Xerosis	Paronychia	Photosensitivity	PPE	Pruritus	Rash
Biotherapy: Other						
Aldesleukin (IL-2; Proleukin®, Novartis Pharmaceuticals)					X	X
Bexarotene (Targretin®, Cardinal Health, Eisai, Ligand Pharmaceuticals)	X				X	X
Denileukin diftitox (Ontak®, Eisai)					X	X
Everolimus (Afinitor®, Novartis Pharmaceuticals)	X				X	X
Interferon (IFN) alfa-2a (Roferon®-A, Roche Pharmaceuticals)	X				X	X
IFN alfa-2b (Intron® A, Schering)	X				X	X
Lenalidomide (Revlimid®, Celgene)	X				X	X
Palifermin (Kepivance®, Amgen)					X	X
Thalidomide (Thalomid®, Celgene)	X				X	X

to 40% in the lowest dose ranges (Mortimer et al., 2003). For patients receiving continuous 5-FU infusions, the incidence of PPE is 42%–82% (Fabian et al., 1990; Wilkes & Doyle, 2005). For patients receiving PLD, the overall incidence of PPE is 13%–50% (Gordon et al., 2000; Mangili et al., 2008; Tanyi et al., 2009; Wilkes & Doyle, 2005). Of the patients receiving PLD at a dose of 50 mg/m^2, 23%–50% develop grade 3 PPE, and 20% develop grade 2 PPE (Gordon et al., 2000; Muggia et al., 1997; Rossi et al., 2007). For patients receiving PLD at dose of 20 mg/m^2, incidence of PPE is 3.4% (Wilkes & Barton-Burke, 2010). PPE can also occur with targeted agents, including sorafenib (34%) and sunitinib (19%) (Helwick, 2009).

Other Skin Reactions

Other skin toxicities occur with less frequency but also contribute to patients' distress and discomfort. Xerosis occurs in patients receiving both chemotherapy and EGFR inhibitors. Incidence of xerosis ranges from 3% to 54.8% (Bianchini et al., 2008; Eaby et al., 2008; Fluhr et al., 2007).

Pruritus is most often reported along with rash, and most of the studies and reports on the management of rash have been done related to the use of EGFR inhibitors. Incidence of rash ranges 8%–52% in patients receiving EGFR inhibitors (Burtness et al., 2009; Lacouture et al., 2006).

Paronychia occurs in 12%–16% of patients receiving EGFR inhibitors and is notable for exquisite tenderness (Burtness et al., 2009; Lacoutoure et al., 2006). Photosensitivity is a known adverse effect of multiple chemotherapeutic agents, as well as EGFR inhibitors (Polovich et al., 2009). Two studies of patients receiving vandetanib reported photosensitivity in 13 of 15 patients in a phase I trial and in 23% of patients with non-small cell lung cancer in a phase II trial (Kong, Fine, Stern, & Turner, 2009).

Prevention

Little data demonstrate the effectiveness of the various approaches used in the attempt to prevent or minimize skin toxicities. However, a number of expert opinion resources recommend some common approaches for prevention. These are discussed in more detail in the review of interventions in the PEP resource. Patient education in general approaches for prevention is recommended, including use of the following strategies.
- Minimize exposure to sunlight or ultraviolet light (Burtness et al., 2009).
- Use sunscreen containing zinc oxide or titanium dioxide to protect skin from the sun (Burtness et al., 2009).
- Avoid temperature extremes to the skin, such as taking long, hot showers or baths, washing dishes, or using cold compresses (Burtness et al., 2009).
- Avoid constrictive clothing, shoes, and jewelry.
- Keep skin moisturized with alcohol-free emollients and use of hypoallergenic skin products (Burtness et al., 2009; Lacouture, Reilly, Gerami, & Guitart, 2008).

- Maintain nail care through
  - Keeping nails short (Dest, 2010)
  - Avoiding exposure to harmful chemicals and detergents (Burtness et al., 2009)
  - Keeping hands and feet moisturized and applying petroleum jelly to the periungual soft tissue frequently (Burtness et al., 2009)
  - Avoiding friction and pressure on the nail fold by wearing shoes that are not too tight (Segaert & Van Cutsem, 2005).

In addition, it is suggested that patients with or at risk for PPE follow these additional recommendations: (a) avoid impact on their feet, such as that from walking, jogging, or aerobics; (b) avoid using tools that require them to squeeze hands on a hard surface, such as kitchen knives or garden tools; and (c) avoid strong massage or rubbing of the area when applying lotions (Lorusso et al., 2007; Markman et al., 2000; Polovich et al., 2009; Swenson & Bell, 2010; Tanyi et al., 2009).

Survivorship and Late Effects

Skin side effects may be episodic, regardless of treatment continuance, and may wax and wane or spontaneously resolve (Lynch et al., 2007). Sensory disturbances, erythema, edema, papulopustular rash, and crusting generally occur early in treatments, with later effects, such as hyperpigmentation, hair changes, paronychia/fissuring, and xerosis, occurring weeks later (Lacouture et al., 2006). Some effects, such as erythema and skin dryness, may persist following treatment discontinuation and may eventually resolve (Herbst et al., 2003). Increased sensitivity to sunlight, telangiectasias, and post-inflammatory hyperpigmentation may occur as long-term side effects or may be permanent (Burtness et al., 2009).

Healthcare providers should remain vigilant, assessing for recurrent symptoms or superinfections secondary to continued use or cyclic recurrence and long-term effects of treatments (Anderson et al., 2009; Burtness et al., 2009). Dermatology referral should be considered as needed (Lacouture, 2007; Perez-Soler & Saltz, 2005).

Assessment and Clinical Measurement Tools

Early and ongoing skin assessments can help to identify and minimize skin reactions. Nurses may identify risk factors by screening the patient's history and medications. In addition to identifying potential skin toxicities associated with the patient's cancer treatment, it is important to determine if the patient has begun any other new medications or over-the-counter agents that may cause these types of reactions as well.

Both objective assessment data (e.g., physical examination of the skin, laboratory and diagnostic testing) and subjective assessment data (e.g., patient-reported symptoms, aggravating and alleviating factors) are needed to ensure that an accurate diagnosis is obtained and appropriate treatment is implemented. Parameters for assessment of skin reactions are outlined in Figure 5-1.

Figure 5-1. Skin and Cutaneous Assessment

Assess risk factors/potential causes of skin/cutaneous effects:

Is the patient receiving therapy associated with skin effects? (See Table 5-2.)	Yes	No
Is the patient using a new product, medication, herbal preparation, vitamin, or another over-the-counter product?	Yes	No

Identify patient symptoms and locations:

Symptom	Location (check sites affected)										
	Armpit	Bra line	Balls of feet	Hands	Heels	Knees	Perito-neum	Thighs	Toes	Waist line	Other
Redness											
Swelling											
Tingling											
Numbness											
Blisters											
Cracks											
Itching											
Fissures											
Rash											
Sores											
Sensitivity to warmth											
Other											

Describe other symptoms/locations:

Is there pain associated with the symptom(s)?	Yes	No

If yes, rate pain:

Mild pain			Moderate pain			Severe pain			Worst
1	2	3	4	5	6	7	8	9	10

Is there anxiety associated with the symptom(s)?	Yes	No

If yes, rate anxiety:

Mild anxiety			Moderate anxiety/distress			Severe anxiety/distress			Worst
1	2	3	4	5	6	7	8	9	10

(Continued on next page)

Figure 5-1. Skin and Cutaneous Assessment *(Continued)*

Are any of these symptoms interfering with:

Ability to function?	Yes	No
Ability to perform normal activities?	Yes	No
Ability to sleep?	Yes	No
Ability to walk?	Yes	No

When were skin changes first experienced?

How did symptoms develop?

Do any of the following aggravate symptoms? (Check all that apply)

☐ Clothing	☐ Friction	☐ Heat	☐ Sunlight	☐ Other

Do any of the following alleviate the symptoms? (Check all that apply)

☐ Scratching	☐ Cool compresses	☐ Lotion	☐ Medications

Pertinent lab and diagnostic testing planned or completed (check if done and date of report)

☐ Skin biopsy (may be needed to assess relation to chemotherapy or infection)	Date:
☐ Punch biopsy and microscopic examination	Date:
☐ Laboratory testing	Date:

Describe:

Note. Based on information from Adams & Nutt, 2006; DeWitt et al., 2007; Economou, 2009; Gordon et al., 1995; Kara et al., 2006; Kimyai-Asadi & Jih, 2002.

Grading scales or measurement tools are often used to assess the severity of the skin toxicity. Table 5-3 outlines a variety of clinical measurement tools for various skin reactions. For several skin reactions (e.g., EGFR inhibitor–induced rash, PPE), toxicity grading is important because it determines the intervention, which could include reducing the drug dose or delaying the treatment. Table 5-4 outlines measurement approaches for PPE and Table 5-5 displays content from the NCI *Common Terminology Criteria for Adverse Events* relevant to skin toxicity. Ongoing assessment is needed to evaluate the effectiveness of interventions (e.g., resolution of signs and symptoms) and modify the interventions and treatment plan, as needed.

Table 5-3. Clinical Measurement Tools

Name of Tool	Number of Items	Applications	Reliability and Validity	Populations	Clinical Utility
Common Terminology Criteria for Adverse Events (NCI CTEP, 2010)	Grading scale: four items	Dry skin PPE Photosensitivity Pruritus/itching Rash: acneform Rash: desquamation	Unknown	Unknown	Often used in clinical trials
Skindex-16 (Chren et al., 2001)	16 items	Symptoms Emotions Functioning	Satisfactory reliability and validity	Patients in dermatology clinics	Used to measure effects of skin disease on patients' quality of life
World Health Organization Grading of PPE (Kara et al., 2006)	Grading scale: four items	PPE symptoms	Unknown	Unknown	Used less frequently in clinical trials
Clinical Trial Grading of PPE (Kara et al., 2006)	Grading scale: four items	PPE symptoms	Unknown	Unknown	Individual grading scales used in specific trials
Dermatology Life Quality Index (Lacouture et al., 2010)	Scored on a scale of 0–30	10 simple questions to assess skin-related QOL	Unknown	Patients with skin disorders	Higher scores indicate more QOL impairment.
Daily diary to document compliance with EGFR inhibitor therapy (Lacouture et al., 2010)	—	—	Unknown	Patients receiving panitumumab	Used to monitor compliance with EGFR inhibitor therapy

(Continued on next page)

Table 5-3. Clinical Measurement Tools (Continued)

Name of Tool	Number of Items	Applications	Reliability and Validity	Populations	Clinical Utility
Rash Incidence Questionnaire (brief) (Jatoi et al., 2008)	Unknown	Unknown	Unknown	Unknown	Used to monitor patients' perception of rash incidence
Photographic evaluation (Scope et al., 2007; Vasconcellos et al., 2009)	Digital photo	—	—	—	Used to document the visual appearance of the rash

EGFR—epidermal growth factor receptor; NCI CTEP—National Cancer Institute Cancer Therapy Evaluation Program; PPE—palmar-plantar erythrodysesthesia; QOL—quality of life

Table 5-4. Grading of Palmar-Plantar Erythrodysesthesia (PPE) Using National Cancer Institute *Common Terminology Criteria for Adverse Events* and Other Grading Systems

Grading System	Grade 1	Grade 2	Grade 3	Grade 4
Clinical grading (Kara et al., 2006)	Numbness, dysesthesia/ paresthesia, tingling, pain-less swelling or erythema	Painful erythe-ma with swell-ing	Moist desqua-mation, ulcer-ation, blistering, severe pain	–
Skin toxicity grade (sorafenib pack-age insert) (Ander-son et al., 2009)	Numbness, dysesthesia, paresthesia, tingling, pain-less swelling, erythema or discomfort of the hands or feet that does not disrupt the patient's normal ADL	Painful ery-thema and swelling of the hands or feet and/or discom-fort affecting the patient's ADL	Moist desqua-mation, ulcer-ation, blistering, or severe pain of the hands or feet or severe discomfort that causes the pa-tient to be un-able to work or perform ADL	–
NCI CTEP CTCAE Version 4.03 June 14, 2010	Minimal skin changes or dermatitis (e.g., erythema, edema, or hy-perkeratosis) without pain	Skin changes (e.g., peeling, blisters, bleed-ing, edema, or hyperkerato-sis) with pain; limiting instru-mental ADL	Severe skin changes (e.g., peeling, blis-ters, bleeding, edema, or hy-perkeratosis) with pain; lim-iting self-care ADL	–
NCI CTEP CTCAE Version 3 2003 (Anderson et al., 2009; Saif et al., 2007)	Minimal skin changes or der-matitis (e.g., er-ythema, peel-ing) with altered sensations (e.g., numb-ness, tingling, burning) that do not interfere with ADL	Skin changes (e.g., peeling, blisters, bleed-ing, edema) present with accompany-ing pain, inter-fering little with ADL. Skin sur-face remains intact.	Ulcerative der-matitis or skin changes with severe pain in-terfering with ADL; tissue breakdown is evident (e.g., peeling, blis-ters, bleeding, edema)	–

(Continued on next page)

Table 5-4. Grading of Palmar-Plantar Erythrodysesthesia (PPE) Using National Cancer Institute *Common Terminology Criteria for Adverse Events* and Other Grading Systems *(Continued)*

Grading System	Grade 1	Grade 2	Grade 3	Grade 4
NCI CTEP CTCAE Version 2 (Drake et al., 2004; Lorusso et al., 2007; Molpus et al., 2004; Rose et al., 2001)	Mild erythema, swelling, or desquamation not interfering with daily activities	Erythema, swelling, or desquamation interfering with daily activities; small blisters or ulceration smaller than 2 cm	Blistering, ulceration, or swelling interfering with daily activities; cannot wear regular clothing	Diffuse or local process causing infectious complications or a bedridden state or hospitalization
NCI CTEP CTCAE Version 1 (Eng et al., 2001; Kara et al., 2006; Mortimer et al., 2003)	Skin changes or dermatitis without pain (i.e., erythema, peeling)	Skin changes with pain, not interfering with function	Skin changes with pain, interfering with function	–
World Health Organization Grading of PPE (Kara et al., 2006)	Dysesthesia/ paresthesia, tingling in hands and feet	Discomfort in holding objects and upon walking; painless swelling or erythema	Painful erythema and swelling of palms and soles, periungual erythema and swelling	Desquamation, ulceration, blistering, severe pain
Clinical grading (Fabian et al., 1990)	Numbness, nail changes, painless swelling	Painful erythema, with or without swelling	Moist desquamation	–

ADL—activities of daily living; NCI CTEP CTCAE—National Cancer Institute Cancer Therapy Evaluation Program *Common Terminology Criteria for Adverse Events*; PPE—palmar-plantar erythrodysesthesia

Note. Grade 0 = normal.

Table 5-5. National Cancer Institute *Common Terminology Criteria for Adverse Events* Categories Relevant to Selected Skin Disorders

Adverse Event	Grade 1 (Mild)	Grade 2 (Moderate)	Grade 3 (Severe)	Grade 4 (Life Threatening)
Rash, acneform	Papules and/or pustules covering < 10% BSA, which may or may not be associated with symptoms of pruritus or tenderness	Papules and/or pustules covering 10%–30% BSA, which may or may not be associated with symptoms of pruritus or tenderness; associated with psychosocial impact; limiting instrumental ADL	Papules and/or pustules covering > 30% BSA, which may or may not be associated with symptoms of pruritus or tenderness; limiting self-care ADL; associated with local superinfection with oral antibiotics indicated	Papules and/or pustules covering any percentage of BSA, which may or may not be associated with symptoms of pruritus or tenderness and are associated with extensive superinfection with IV antibiotics indicated; life-threatening consequences
Rash, maculopapular	Macules/papules covering < 10% BSA with or without symptoms (e.g., pruritus, burning, tightness)	Macules/papules covering 10%–30% BSA with or without symptoms (e.g., pruritus, burning, tightness); limiting instrumental ADL	Macules/papules covering > 30% BSA with or without associated symptoms; limiting self-care ADL	–
Photosensitivity	Painless erythema and erythema covering < 10% BSA	Tender erythema covering 10%–30% BSA	Erythema covering > 30% BSA and erythema with blistering; photosensitivity; oral corticosteroid therapy indicated; pain control indicated (e.g., narcotics or NSAIDs)	Life-threatening consequences; urgent intervention indicated

(Continued on next page)

Table 5-5. National Cancer Institute *Common Terminology Criteria for Adverse Events* Categories Relevant to Selected Skin Disorders *(Continued)*

Adverse Event	Grade 1 (Mild)	Grade 2 (Moderate)	Grade 3 (Severe)	Grade 4 (Life Threatening)
Pruritus/ itching	Mild or localized; topical intervention indicated	Intense or widespread; intermittent; skin changes from scratching (e.g., edema, papulation, excoriations, lichenification, oozing/crusts); oral intervention indicated; limiting instrumental ADL	Intense or widespread; constant; limiting self-care ADL or sleep; oral corticosteroid or immunosuppressive therapy indicated	–
Xerosis/dry skin	Covering < 10% BSA and not associated erythema or pruritus	Covering 10%–30% BSA and associated with erythema or pruritus; limiting instrumental ADL	Covering > 30% BSA and associated with pruritus; limiting self-care ADL	–

ADL—activities of daily living; BSA—body surface area; NSAIDs—nonsteroidal anti-inflammatory drugs

Note. Grade 5 = death.

From *Common Terminology Criteria for Adverse Events* [v.4.03], by National Cancer Institute Cancer Therapy Evaluation Program, 2010. Retrieved from http://evs.nci.nih.gov/ftp1/CTCAE/CTCAE_4.03_2010-06-14_QuickReference_8.5x11.pdf.

References

Adams, D.H., & Nutt, T. (2006). A case report and discussion of cetuximab-induced folliculitis. *American Journal of Clinical Dermatology, 7,* 333–336.

Anderson, R., Jatoi, A., Robert, C., Wood, L.S., Keating, K.N., & Lacouture, M.E. (2009). Search for evidence-based approaches for the prevention and palliation of hand-foot skin reaction (HFSR) caused by the multikinase inhibitors (MKIs). *Oncologist, 14,* 291–302. doi:10.1634/theoncologist.2008-0237

Bianchini, D., Jayanth, A., Chua, Y.J., & Cunningham, D. (2008). Epidermal growth factor receptor inhibitor-related skin toxicity: Mechanisms, treatment, and its potential role as a predictive marker. *Clinical Colorectal Cancer, 7,* 33–43.

Burtness, B., Anadkat, M., Basti, S., Hughes, M., Lacouture, M.E., McClure, J.S., ... Spencer, S. (2009). NCCN task force report: Management of dermatologic and other toxicities associated with EGFR inhibition in patients with cancer. *Journal of the National Comprehensive Cancer Network, 7*(Suppl. 1), S5–S21.

Chren, M.M., Lasek, R.J., Sahay, A.P., & Sands, L.P. (2001). Measurement properties of Skindex-16: A brief quality of life measure for patients with skin diseases. doi:10.1007/s102270000010

de Noronha e Menezes, N.M., Lima, R., Moreira, A., Varela, P., Barroso, A., Baptista, A., & Parente, B. (2009). Description and management of cutaneous side effects during erlotinib and cetuximab treatment in lung and colorectal cancer patients: A prospective and descriptive study of 19 patients. *European Journal of Dermatology, 19,* 248–251. doi:10.1684/ejd.2009.0650

Dest, V.M. (2010). Systemic therapy–induced skin reactions. In M.L. Haas & G.J. Moore-Higgs (Eds.), *Principles of skin care and the oncology patient* (pp. 141–166). Pittsburgh, PA: Oncology Nursing Society.

DeWitt, C.A., Siroy, A.E., & Stone, S.P. (2007). Acneiform eruptions associated with epidermal growth factor receptor–targeted chemotherapy. *Journal of the American Academy of Dermatology, 56,* 500–505. doi:10.1016/j.jaad.2006.06.046

Drake, R.D., Lin, W.M., King, M., Farrar, D., Miller, D.S., & Coleman, R.L. (2004). Oral dexamethasone attenuates Doxil-induced palmar-plantar erythrodysesthesias in patients with recurrent gynecologic malignancies. *Gynecologic Oncology, 94,* 320–324. doi:10.1016/j.ygyno.2004.05.027

Dubakiene, R., & Kupriene, M. (2006). Scientific problems of photosensitivity. *Medicina, 42,* 619–624.

Eaby, B., Culkin, A., & Lacouture, M.E. (2008). An interdisciplinary consensus on managing skin reactions associated with human epidermal growth factor receptor inhibitors. *Clinical Journal of Oncology Nursing, 12,* 283–290. doi:10.1188/08.CJON.283-290

Economou, D. (2009). Pruritus. In S. Newton, M. Hickey, & J. Marrs (Eds.), *Oncology nursing advisor: A comprehensive guide to clinical practice* (pp. 385–386). St. Louis, MO: Elsevier Mosby.

Esper, P., Gale, D., & Muehlbauer, P. (2007). What kind of rash is it?: Deciphering the dermatologic toxicities of biologic and targeted therapies. *Clinical Journal of Oncology Nursing, 11,* 659–666. doi:10.1188/07.CJON.659-666

Fabian, C.J., Molina, R., Slavik, M., Dahlberg, S., Giri, S., & Stephens, R. (1990). Pyridoxine therapy for palmar-plantar erythrodysesthesia associated with continuous 5-fluorouracil infusion. *Investigational New Drugs, 8,* 57–63.

Fluhr, J.W., Miteva, M., Primavera, G., Ziemer, M., Elsner, P., & Berardesca, E. (2007). Functional assessment of a skin care system in patients on chemotherapy. *Skin Pharmacology and Physiology, 20,* 253–259. doi:10.1159/000104423

Gordon, A.N., Granai, C.O., Rose, P.G., Hainsworth, J., Lopez, A., Weissman, C., … Sharpington, T. (2000). Phase II study of liposomal doxorubicin in platinum- and paclitaxel-refractory epithelial ovarian cancer. *Journal of Clinical Oncology, 18,* 3093–3100. Retrieved from http://jco.ascopubs.org/content/18/17/3093.long

Gordon, K.B., Tajuddin, A., Guitart, J., Kuzel, T.M., Eramo, L.R., & Von Roenn, J. (1995). Hand-foot syndrome associated with liposome-encapsulated doxorubicin therapy. *Cancer, 75,* 2169–2173. doi:10.1002/1097-0142(19950415)75:8<2169::AID-CNCR2820750822>3.0.CO;2-H

Helwick, C. (2009). Information for patients. HER2+ early breast cancer: Understanding adjuvant treatment. *Oncology, 23*(11, Suppl. Nurse Ed.), 8a–8b.

Heo, Y.S., Chang, H.M., Kim, T.W., Ryu, M., Ahn, J., Kim, S.B., … Kang, Y. (2004). Hand-foot syndrome in patients treated with capecitabine-containing combination chemotherapy. *Journal of Clinical Pharmacology, 44,* 1166–1172.

Herbst, R.S., LoRusso, P.M., Purdom, M., & Ward, D. (2003). Dermatologic side effects associated with gefitinib therapy: Clinical experience and management. *Clinical Lung Cancer, 4,* 366–369. doi:10.3816/CLC.2003.n.016

Jatoi, A., Rowland, K., Sloan, J.A., Gross, H.M., Fishkin, P.A., Kahanic, S.P., … Loprinzi, C.L. (2008). Tetracycline to prevent epidermal growth factor receptor inhibitor-induced skin rashes: Results of a placebo-controlled trial from the North Central Cancer Treatment Group (N03CB). *Cancer, 113,* 847–853. doi:10.1002/cncr.23621

Jia, Y., Lacouture, M.E., Su, X., & Wu, S. (2009). Risk of skin rash associated with erlotinib in cancer patients: A meta-analysis. *Journal of Supportive Oncology, 7,* 211–217.

Kara, I.O., Sahin, B., & Erkisi, M. (2006). Palmar-plantar erythrodysesthesia due to docetaxel-capecitabine therapy is treated with vitamin E without dose reduction. *Breast, 15,* 413–423. doi:10.1016/j.breast.2005.07.007

Kimyai-Asadi, A., & Jih, M.H. (2002). Follicular toxic effects of chimeric anti-epidermal growth factor receptor antibody cetuximab used to treat human solid tumors. *Archives of Dermatology, 138,* 129–131. doi:10.1001/archderm.138.1.129

Kong, H.H., Fine, H.A., Stern, J.B., & Turner, M.L. (2009). Cutaneous pigmentation after photosensitivity induced by vandetanib therapy. *Archives of Dermatology, 145,* 923–925. doi:10.1001/archdermatol.2009.177

Lacouture, M.E. (2007). Insights into the pathophysiology and management of dermatologic toxicities to EGFR-targeted therapies in colorectal cancer. *Cancer Nursing, 30*(4, Suppl. 1), S17–S26. doi:10.1097/01.NCC.0000281758.85704.9b

Lacouture, M.E., Basti, S., Patel, J., & Benson, A., III. (2006). The SERIES clinic: An interdisciplinary approach to the management of toxicities of EGFR inhibitors. *Journal of Supportive Oncology, 4,* 236–238.

Lacouture, M.E., Maitland, M.L., Segaert, S., Setser, A., Baran, R., Fox, L.P., ... Trotti, A. (2010). A proposed EGFR inhibitor dermatologic adverse event-specific grading scale from the MASCC Skin Toxicity Study Group. *Supportive Care in Cancer, 18,* 509–522. doi:10.1007/s00520-009-0744-x

Lacouture, M.E., Reilly, L.M., Gerami, P., & Guitart, J. (2008). Hand foot skin reaction in cancer patients treated with the multikinase inhibitors sorafenib and sunitinib. *Annals of Oncology, 19,* 1955–1961. doi:10.1093/annonc/mdn389

Lorusso, D., Di Stefano, A., Carone, V., Fagotti, A., Pisconti, S., & Scambia, G. (2007). Pegylated liposomal doxorubicin-related palmar-plantar erythrodysesthesia (hand-foot syndrome). *Annals of Oncology, 18,* 1159–1164. doi:10.1093/annonc/mdl477

Lynch, T.J., Jr., Kim, E.S., Eaby, B., Garey, J., West, D.P., & Lacouture, M.E. (2007). Epidermal growth factor receptor inhibitor-associated cutaneous toxicities: An evolving paradigm in clinical management. *Oncologist, 12,* 610–621. doi:10.1634/theoncologist.12-5-610

Mangili, G., Petrone, M., Gentile, C., De Marzi, P., Viganò, R., & Rabaiotti, E. (2008). Prevention strategies in palmar-plantar erythrodysesthesia onset: The role of regional cooling. *Gynecologic Oncology, 108,* 332–335. doi:10.1016/j.ygyno.2007.10.021

Markman, M., Kennedy, A., Webster, K., Peterson, G., Kulp, B., & Belinson, J. (2000). Phase 2 trial of liposomal doxorubicin (40 mg/m^2) in platinum/paclitaxel-refractory ovarian and fallopian tube cancers and primary carcinoma of the peritoneum. *Gynecologic Oncology, 78*(3, Pt. 1), 369–372. doi:10.1006/gyno.2000.5921

Melosky, B., Burkes, R., Rayson, D., Alcindor, T., Shear, N., & Lacouture, M. (2009). Management of skin rash during EGFR-targeted monoclonal antibody treatment for gastrointestinal malignancies: Canadian recommendations. *Current Oncology, 16*(1), 16–26.

Micantonio, T., Fargnoli, M.C., Ricevuto, E., Ficorella, C., Marchetti, P., & Peris, K. (2005). Efficacy of treatment with tetracyclines to prevent acneiform eruption secondary to cetuximab therapy. *Archives of Dermatology, 141,* 1173–1174. doi:10.1001/archderm.141.9.1173

Molinari, E., De Quatrebarbes, J., André, T., & Aractingi, S. (2005). Cetuximab-induced acne. *Dermatology, 211,* 330–333. doi:10.1159/000088502

Molpus, K.L., Anderson, L.B., Craig, C.L., & Pulee, J.G. (2004). The effect of regional cooling on toxicity associated with intravenous infusion of pegylated liposomal doxorubicin in recurrent ovarian carcinoma. *Gynecologic Oncology, 93,* 513–516.

Mortimer, J.E., Lauman, M.K., Tan, B., Dempsey, C.L., Shillington, A.C., & Hutchins, K.S. (2003). Pyridoxine treatment and prevention of hand-and-foot syndrome in patients receiving capecitabine. *Journal of Oncology Pharmacy Practice, 9,* 161–166. doi:10.1191/1078155203jp116oa

Muggia, F.M., Hainsworth, J.D., Jeffers, S., Miller, P., Groshen, S., Tan, M., ... Liang, L.J. (1997). Phase II study of liposomal doxorubicin in refractory ovarian cancer: Antitumor activity and toxicity modification by liposomal encapsulation. *Journal of Clinical Oncology, 15,* 987–993.

National Cancer Institute Cancer Therapy Evaluation Program. (2010). *Common terminology criteria for adverse events* [v.4.03]. Retrieved from http://evs.nci.nih.gov/ftp1/CTCAE/About.html

Oishi, K. (2008). Clinical approaches to minimize rash associated with EGFR inhibitors. *Oncology Nursing Forum, 35,* 103–111. doi:10.1188/08.ONS.103-111

Perez-Soler, R., & Saltz, L. (2005). Cutaneous adverse effects with HER1/EGFR-targeted agents: Is there a silver lining? *Journal of Clinical Oncology, 23,* 5235–5246. doi:10.1200/JCO.2005.00.6916

Polovich, M., Whitford, J.M., & Olsen, M. (Eds.). (2009). *Chemotherapy and biotherapy guidelines and recommendations for practice* (3rd ed.). Pittsburgh, PA: Oncology Nursing Society.

Rose, P.G., Maxson, J.H., Fusco, N., Mossbruger, K., & Rodriguez, M. (2001). Liposomal doxorubicin in ovarian, peritoneal, and tubal carcinoma: A retrospective comparative study of single agent dosages. *Gynecologic Oncology, 82,* 323–328. doi:10.1006/gyno.2001.6272

Rossi, D., Alessandroni, P., Catalano, V., Giordani, P., Fedeli, S.L., Fedeli, A., ... Catalano, G. (2007). Safety profile and activity of lower capecitabine dose in patients with metastatic breast cancer. *Clinical Breast Cancer, 7,* 857–860.

Saif, M.W., Elfiky, A., & Diasio, R. (2007). Hand-foot syndrome variant in a dihydropyrimidine dehydrogenase-deficient patient treated with capecitabine. *Clinical Colorectal Cancer, 6,* 219–223.

Schwartzentruber, D.J. (2000). Interleukin-2: Clinical applications: Principles of administration and management of side effects. In S.A. Rosenberg (Ed.), *Principles and practice of the biologic therapy of cancer* (3rd ed., pp. 32–50). Philadelphia, PA: Lippincott Williams & Wilkins.

Scope, A., Agero, A.L., Dusza, S.W., Myskowski, P.L., Lieb, J.A., Saltz, L., ... Halpern, A.C. (2007). Randomized double-blind trial of prophylactic oral minocycline and topical tazarotene for cetuximab-associated acne-like eruption. *Journal of Clinical Oncology, 25,* 5390–5396. doi:10.1200/JCO.2007.12.6987

Segaert, S., & Van Cutsem, E. (2005). Clinical signs, pathophysiology and management of skin toxicity during therapy with epidermal growth factor receptor inhibitors. *Annals of Oncology, 16,* 1425–1433. doi:10.1093/annonc/mdi279

Swenson, K.K., & Bell, E.M. (2010). Hand-foot syndrome related to liposomal doxorubicin. *Oncology Nursing Forum, 37,* 137–139. doi:10.1188/10.ONF.137-139

Tanyi, J.L., Smith, J.A., Ramos, L., Parker, C.L., Munsell, M.F., & Wolf, J.K. (2009). Predisposing risk factors for palmar-plantar erythrodesia when using liposomal doxyrubicin to treat recurrent ovarian cancer. *Gynecologic Oncology, 114,* 219–224. doi:10.1016/j.ygyno.2009.04.007

Viale, P.H. (2010). Incorporating new data on colorectal cancer into nursing practice. *Clinical Journal of Oncology Nursing, 14,* 92–100. doi:10.1188/10.CJON.92-100

Wilkes, G.M., & Barton-Burke, M. (2010). *Oncology nursing drug handbook.* Sudbury, MA: Jones and Bartlett.

Wilkes, G.M., & Doyle, D. (2005). Palmar-plantar erythrodysesthesia. *Clinical Journal of Oncology Nursing, 9,* 103–106. doi:10.1188/05.CJON.103-106

Wright, L.G. (2006). Maculopapular skin rashes associated with high-dose chemotherapy: Prevalence and risk factors. *Oncology Nursing Forum, 33,* 1095–1103. doi:10.1188/06.ONF.1095-1103

Case Study

Q.W. is a 63-year-old Asian American female who works as an officer in a small bank and has never smoked. She was diagnosed with non-small cell lung cancer with bone metastasis after presenting with complaints of a cough and low back pain. At diagnosis, her Eastern Cooperative Oncology Group performance status was 1. She initially received a chemotherapy regimen of cisplatin and pemetrexed. After two cycles of therapy, a positron-emission tomography (PET) scan showed that the primary lung tumor had increased in size since her initial evaluation.

Because her tumor was positive for an EGFR mutation and negative for Kirsten rat sarcoma viral oncogene, she was started on the EGFR inhibitor erlotinib 150 mg daily by mouth as a single agent. She was counseled that she might develop skin problems, such as a rash on her face and upper body or redness and pain around her nails, from the therapy. She was advised to wash her skin with a mild soap, such as Dove® (Unilever), and apply a skin moisturizer, such as Eucerin® (Beiersdorf, Inc.) daily. She also was instructed to notify the clinic if she developed any skin problems. She was told that development of a rash might indicate that the therapy was effective, so it was important to control a rash so that her therapy did not need to be decreased or stopped.

Eight days after the start of the erlotinib, Q.W. began to develop red patches on her face. She notified the clinic and was told to continue the skin care as prescribed and to monitor the rash. Two days later, the patient reported that the number of red areas on her face had increased, and she had red areas on her shoulders, back, and chest. She reported that the spots on her face were burning and that her scalp, back, and chest were itching. She was instructed to continue her skin care and to come to the clinic the following day for evaluation.

The following day, Q.W. was examined in the clinic and found to have confluent erythematous papules and small perifollicular pustules on her cheeks, nose, chin, shoulders, upper back, and upper chest. Comedones were not identified. Q.W. expressed concern that she found the rash very embarrassing and was afraid she might have to cut back or stop working if the rash was not controlled. The EGFR inhibitor–induced rash was classified as a grade II according to the *Common Terminology Criteria for Adverse Events*. She said that her 16-year-old grandson had commented that her skin looked worse than his acne, and he recommended some acne cleanser and lotion that had worked for him. Q.W. asked if these products might help her rash. The oncology nurse explained that her rash was not the same as acne and that acne medications might actually make the skin problems worse.

Q.W. was given topical pimecrolimus (Elidel®, Novartis Pharmaceuticals) to apply to the rash and started on doxycycline 50 mg twice daily. She was told to continue the rest of the previously recommended skin care regimen. She was also told that she could use cosmetics to hide the rash on the exposed parts of her face and upper body. She was advised to call the clinic if the rash spread or worsened. She was told that she would be referred to a dermatologist if the rash worsened.

A follow-up examination 10 days later showed significant improvement in the erythema, a reduction in the number of lesions on her face, back, and chest, and a decrease in the size of the lesions. Q.W. was continuing to work and was happy with the improvement in the rash.

Approximately five weeks after starting the erlotinib, Q.W. again contacted her clinic nurse to complain of redness and tenderness around the nails of her index and middle fingers on her right hand. The nurse advised her that this was another expected side effect of the erlotinib. The nurse told her to soak her fingers in warm, soapy water for 15 minutes four times a day. If she noticed the redness and pain spreading beyond the area immediately around the nail or pus coming from the area, she should contact the nurse. After one week, the pain and redness around her nails resolved.

Eight weeks after beginning erlotinib, Q.W. had a PET scan, which showed that the primary lung tumor had decreased by approximately 50%. She had no new evidence of disease, experienced no other cutaneous toxicities, and remained on the erlotinib therapy.

Skin Reactions

AUTHORS
Jeanene (Gigi) Robison, MSN, RN, AOCN®, Therese Carpizo, MSN, RN, AOCN®,
Julie Carlson, MSN, RN, APN, AOCNS®, Ann Fuhrman, BSN, RN, OCN®,
Denise Portz, BSN, RN, OCN®, Gary Shelton, MSN, ANP-BC, RN, AOCNP®,
and Loretta A. Williams, PhD, RN, AOCN®
LIBRARIAN: Mark Vrabel, MLS, AHIP, ELS
ONS STAFF: Kristen Fessele, RN, MSN, ANP-BC, AOCN®, Margaret Irwin, PhD, RN, MN

What interventions are effective for the prevention and management of rash, xerosis, pruritus, palmar-plantar erythrodysesthesia (PPE), and photosensitivity associated with cancer treatment?

Overview

Interventions for the prevention and management of skin reactions associated with chemotherapy and biotherapy have varied related to the specific type of skin toxicity addressed as well as the type of intervention. Table 5-1 in the book chapter content shows the evidence of intervention type and application to the specific skin effect reviewed here. Interventions have included local or regional treatments, topical agents, systemic treatments, and other interventions. The evidence is summarized and grouped according to intervention types and agents and specific skin toxicity involved. Much of the evidence exists only in the form of case series or individual case studies. In addition, many of the interventions reported are combinations of several treatment types, which makes the process of determining the impact of individual treatments challenging.

Recommended for Practice

Interventions for which effectiveness has been demonstrated by strong evidence from rigorously conducted studies, meta-analyses, or systematic reviews and for which expectation of harms is small compared with the benefits

No interventions are recommended as of February 2010.

Likely to Be Effective

Interventions for which effectiveness has been demonstrated by supportive evidence from a single rigorously conducted controlled trial, consistent supportive evidence from well-designed controlled trials using small samples, or guidelines developed from evidence and supported by expert opinion

There are no interventions as of February 2010.

Benefits Balanced With Harms

Interventions for which clinicians and patients should weigh the beneficial and harmful effects according to individual circumstances and priorities

There are no interventions as of February 2010.

Effectiveness Not Established

Interventions for which insufficient or conflicting data or data of inadequate quality currently exist, with no clear indication of harm

LOCAL AND REGIONAL TREATMENTS

A variety of local and regional interventions have been used for preventing and treating many skin reactions to chemotherapy and biotherapy agents. One case study reported on local treatment of epidermal growth factor receptor (EGFR) inhibitor–induced rash using a combination of local agents and systemic treatment with antibiotics. Several studies have examined the effect of regional cooling on PPE. Results in this area are mixed. Many different topical agents have been used to treat EGFR inhibitor–induced rash, PPE, xerosis, pruritus, and paronychia.

Local Treatments for EGFR Inhibitor–Induced Rash

Combination therapy: acetic acid, salicylic acid, and local and systemic antibiotics: A case report of a 52-year-old white male with stage IV colon cancer on cetuximab as adjuvant to 5-fluorouracil (5-FU), leucovorin, and irinotecan described a papulopustular rash on the face, neck, chest, back, and scalp. Treatment with oral minocycline 100 mg twice daily, adapalene 0.1% gel twice daily, and dilute acetic acid soaks plus mupirocin cream three to four times per day to facial and scalp encrustations, with salicylic acid shampoo, resulted in significant improvement to erythema and crusting (DeWitt, Siroy, & Stone, 2007).

Regional Treatment for PPE

Cooling, regional: The evidence related to the potential benefits and harms of regional cooling as an intervention is unclear because results are mixed. In one retrospective chart review of 330 women with gynecologic cancers who received pegylated liposomal doxorubicin (PLD), the proportion of patients with PPE was significantly higher among those patients who used a regional cooling mechanism as compared to those who did not (39% versus 26%, p = 0.0067) (Tanyi et al., 2009). Additional studies have reviewed the effectiveness of this intervention to prevent PPE, and results demonstrated a decrease in the incidence and severity of PPE symptoms with regional cooling (Mangili et al., 2006, 2008; Molpus, Anderson, Craig, & Pulee, 2004; Tedjarati, Sayer, Boulware, & Apte, 2006). In one case study, regional cooling was effective in treating PPE symptoms (Zimmerman et al., 1994).

TOPICAL AGENTS

Topical agents studied or reported as case studies include antiseptics, antibiotics, dimethyl sulfoxide (DMSO), an immune modulator, steroids, retinoids, and petroleum- or urea-based emollients. These interventions were evaluated for the prevention or treatment of EGFR inhibitor–induced rash, PPE, xerosis, and pruritus.

Antiseptics, Topical

Three reports were found regarding the use of topical antiseptic agents, two on the use of benzoyl peroxide alone or in combination with a retinoid in the treatment of EGFR inhibitor–induced rash and one using Bag Balm® (Dairy Association Inc.) in the treatment of PPE (Chin et al., 2001). Bag Balm, which is usually categorized as an emollient, is included in the antiseptics section because it contains hydroxyquinoline sulfate, which has antiseptic properties.

Two case reports discussed the effectiveness of benzoyl peroxide. One case study (DeWitt et al., 2007) discussed a patient who received EGFR inhibitor therapy and developed a rash. This patient's rash significantly improved with 0.1% adapalene gel applied nightly and benzoyl peroxide 4% gel applied in the mornings. Another case study (Molinari, De Quatrebarbes, André, & Aractingi, 2005) reported a case of a patient who received EGFR inhibitor therapy and developed a rash and experienced benefit with benzoyl peroxide. In contrast, in the 2009 National Comprehensive Cancer Network (NCCN) Task Force Report on the management of skin toxicities associated with EGFR inhibitor therapy, NCCN suggested that most conventional topical anti-acne treatments, including benzoyl peroxide, are not indicated to treat the skin rash (Burtness et al., 2009).

A study to evaluate the effectiveness of Bag Balm was conducted on 39 patients receiving various chemotherapy agents, including PLD and continuous 5-FU. (Bag Balm, a topical petroleum-lanolin–based ointment, contains an antiseptic ingredient, hydroxyquinoline sulfate, and is intended for veterinary use to soothe animal udders.) Thirteen patients developed PPE, and the application of Bag Balm three times a day resulted in improvement of PPE appearance (Chin et al., 2001).

Antibiotics, Topical

A variety of case reports and series have discussed the use of topical antibiotics for the treatment of EGFR inhibitor–induced rash and paronychia.

Use of topical antibiotics in EGFR inhibitor–induced rash: Seven reports or case series that involved the use of topical antibiotics for the management of EGFR inhibitor–induced skin toxicities were found.

1. Several researchers reported a case series of 30 patients who received cetuximab. Topical antibiotics (mostly clindamycin 1% and erythromycin) were used in two patients with grade 3 and five patients with grade 2 rash, in combination with vitamin K_1 cream. This treatment resulted in partial resolution of the rash (Ocvirk & Rebersek, 2008).

2. Several researchers described a case series of patients who received cetuximab (N = 20). The rash was treated with erythromycin 4% gel or phosphate clindamycin oil in cream. Four patients who developed a grade 3 rash also received doxycycline 100 mg orally. The rash in all patients was completely resolved at the eight-week follow-up visit (Racca et al., 2008).

3. One case study described a patient who was receiving cetuximab and developed a rash. Treatment with topical clindamycin 1% gel resulted in near resolution of the EGFR inhibitor–induced rash (Adams & Nutt, 2006).

4. Other authors have described case reports of two patients who received cetuximab and developed a rash. The rash in the first patient was treated with topical metronidazole 0.75% gel and oral isotretinoin 30 mg, and completely resolved. The rash in the second patient was treated with topical metronidazole 0.75% gel and oral isotretinoin 40 mg. The rash worsened, and therapy was changed to 1% erythromycin, 2% triclosan in unguentum leniens, and oral isotretinoin 40 mg. The skin eruptions markedly improved (Gutzmer, Werfel, Mao, Kapp, & Elsner, 2005).

5. In one case report, a patient was receiving cetuximab and developed a rash. The patient was given prophylactic oral antibiotics, and topical 5% fusidic acid cream was applied to the rash. The result was a partial resolution of the rash (Micantonio et al., 2005).

6. Other researchers used a case series of patients receiving EGFR inhibitors, including gefitinib and cetuximab. In six patients, the rash was treated with fusidic acid cream as monotherapy or in combination with another treatment. A complete resolution of the rash was obtained on one patient, and a partial resolution was obtained in five patients. In four patients, topical erythromycin 4% solution was applied to the rash as monotherapy or combined with another treatment. This resulted in partial resolution of the rash for two patients, no improvement for one patient, and not reported for one patient. In two patients, topical erythromycin 4% solution and systemic fusidic acid was administered to prevent rash, and this was successful (Jacot et al., 2004).

7. Another case report described a patient who was receiving cetuximab and developed a rash. The combined interventions of topical clindamycin phosphate solution and triamcinolone acetonide cream, along with discontinuation of the EGFR inhibitor therapy, resulted in resolution of the rash. When the EGFR inhibitor therapy was resumed, the skin eruptions were worse, despite the use of topical treatment (Kimyai-Asadi & Jih, 2002).

Two notable sources described the use of topical antibiotics. Tan and Chan (2009) compiled the results of multiple case reports, case series, and randomized controlled trials related to the treatment of skin toxicities associated with EGFR inhibitor therapy. In their systematic review of the literature, they concluded that topical antibiotics appear to be more effective than most other treatment options for milder skin reactions. However, they emphasized that topical antibiotics are commonly combined with other agents, which makes it difficult to draw firm conclusions about which specific agents were effective. This review was greatly limited by the small amount and varied quality of the available evidence (Tan & Chan, 2009). In the NCCN Task Force Report, authors noted that the use of topical antibiotics to treat EGFR inhibitor–induced rash is based more on preference and clinical experience than on data from clinical trials (Burtness et al., 2009).

Use of topical antibiotics in EGFR inhibitor–induced paronychia: In case reports of the treatment of paronychia, topical antibiotics were combined with other topical and/or systemic treatments. Studies evaluating the effectiveness of topical antibiotics for paronychia have mixed results. One case series review was found in which paronychia was managed with a combination of topical and systemic antibiotics and steroids. Boucher, Davidson, Mirakhur, Goldber, and Heymann (2002) reported a case study where self-treatment of paronychia with neomycin ointment and bleach was ineffective.

Suh, Kindler, Medenica, and Lacouture (2006) reported on one patient who was receiving cetuximab (an EGFR inhibitor) and developed paronychia. The patient was treated with topical mupirocin twice daily and cephalexin 500 mg four times a day for 10 days, with no symptomatic improvement. The EGFR inhibitor treatment was also stopped. Doxycycline 100 mg twice a day was then initiated. After six weeks, this treatment resulted in complete resolution of paronychia and allowed the patient to resume previously limited daily living activities (Suh et al., 2006).

Fox (2007) reported a review of several case reports of the management of patients experiencing EGFR inhibitor–induced paronychia and created a table of interventions. Boucher and colleagues (2002) managed the paronychia for one patient using triamcinolone ointment and nystatin, and the result was partially effective. Nakano and Nakamura (2003) reported on three patients who developed paronychia due to gefitinib for advanced lung cancer. All three patients were treated with topical and systemic antibiotics, which were found to be ineffective. Lee and colleagues (2004) managed the paronychia related to gefitinib with topical antibiotics, and the symptoms of paronychia improved.

DMSO, Topical Use for PPE

One case report discussed two patients who received PLD (50 mg/m^2 every four weeks). The patients developed grade 3 PPE after three cycles of PLD and were treated with topical 99% DMSO four times daily for 14 days. Their PPE symptoms resolved over a period of one to three weeks (Lopez et al., 1999).

Emollients and Moisturizers

A number of studies and case reports were found that reported on the use of emollients and moisturizers in the management of xerosis, pruritus, EGFR inhibitor–induced rash, and PPE. Two reports examined and reported on the management of general skin toxicity effects. One study reported on the effects of a colloidal oatmeal lotion (Alexandrescu, Vaillant, & Dasanu, 2007). Other agents used were either urea- or petroleum-based products, and in most cases, treatment with these products was combined with other local and systemic therapies. In one study, topical treatment was combined with systemic antibiotics as well as topical steroids (Lacouture et al., 2010). In another report, emollients were used in combination with pyridoxine (Saif, Elfiky, & Diasio, 2007). Two reports attempted to examine the effectiveness for prevention of skin toxicities in general (Lacouture et al., 2010; Pendharkar & Goyal, 2004).

Use of Emollients and Moisturizers for General Skin Toxicities, Xerosis, and Pruritus

Colloidal oatmeal lotion: An open-label study evaluated 11 patients receiving EGFR and kinase inhibitor therapy experiencing cutaneous reactions including asymptomatic; erythematous rash and itching; and confluent lesions, tenderness, and deep ulcerations. Severe xerosis was treated with colloidal oatmeal lotion three times a day for seven days. All of the patients had a response, and 60% of the patients had a complete response (Alexandrescu et al., 2007).

Urea- and petroleum-based products: In a case series of 31 patients with metastatic colorectal cancer (CRC) treated with cetuximab, 17 patients experienced dry, itchy skin. All alcohol-containing skin products were discontinued. Oil in water or other hydrating products, including those containing 2%–5% urea, proved "effective" (Ocvirk & Cencelj, 2009).

In another case series, 34 patients who were being treated for metastatic CRC and receiving cetuximab and irinotecan were enrolled in a phase II multisite, uncontrolled clinical trial. Dry skin was treated with ointment-based moisturizing emollients. All dermatologic events were reversible within four weeks of treatment discontinuation (Racca et al., 2008).

In a nonrandomized, non–double-blind controlled study of 30 patients diagnosed with gastrointestinal, breast, prostate, or lung cancers or lymphoma, the patients were treated with a slightly acidic pH cleanser and emollient for dry, sensitive skin, SebaMed® Anti-Dry Wash Emulsion and Hydrating Body Lotion (Thompson and Grace Pharmaceuticals).

The control group received water only. In the experimental group, transepidermal water loss was significantly reduced, stratum corneum hydration was increased, skin surface lipids were increased, and skin pH values did not change significantly. A significant gradual reduction in all skin symptoms, including dryness, itching, erythema, and rash, were seen over the three-week course of treatment (p < 0.001) (Fluhr et al., 2007).

Use of moisturizer in combination with steroids and antibiotics: In a phase II, open-label, randomized trial, a total of 95 patients with metastatic CRC treated with panitumumab were randomly assigned to a preemptive arm or reactive arm to compare the effectiveness of prevention of skin toxicities consisting of daily skin moisturizer, use of sunscreen, topical 1% hydrocortisone cream daily, and oral doxycycline 100 mg twice a day beginning one day prior to the start of panitumumab. The reactive arm received any treatment that the investigator deemed necessary to manage emergent skin toxicities. The results revealed a 29% incidence of skin toxicities in the preemptive arm as compared to a 69% incidence in the reactive group (Lacouture et al., 2010).

In one case report, a patient was treated with Iressa® (AstraZeneca), which was dosed blindly at either 250 mg or 500 mg daily. The patient experienced scaling skin, which was treated with emollients and minocycline 100 mg daily. Dryness was resolved (Van Doorn, Kirtschig, Scheffer, Stoof, & Giaccone, 2002).

Use of emollients and moisturizers for PPE: Two studies and two case reports were found that reported on the use of topical emollients or moisturizers related to PPE. One study examined the use of a urea-based product, and one reported on a petroleum-based product. In these cases the topical agent was used in combination with pyridoxine and dose reduction of the cancer treatment regimen. These studies involved very small numbers of patients. In the case reports, improvement in PPE appeared to be substantially affected by treatment dose modification rather than the topical treatment.

In a nonrandomized, noncontrolled study, 13 patients with cancer received capecitabine and developed PPE. They were treated with Cotaryl® (Spectra), containing 12.5% urea, twice a day. These patients experienced decreased levels of skin desquamation and pain and increased comfort. Seven patients were treated prophylactically with the same preparation; five did not develop PPE, and two patients experienced grade 1 PPE (Pendharkar & Goyal, 2004).

A study to evaluate the effect of Bag Balm, a topical, petroleum-based ointment with antiseptic properties, was conducted on 39 patients receiving various chemotherapy agents, including PLD and continuous 5-FU. Thirteen patients developed PPE, and the application of Bag Balm three times a day resulted in improvement of PPE appearance (Chin et al., 2001).

A report of two cases demonstrated the impact of modifying the chemotherapy regimen. The first case report documented PPE treatment in a patient with stage IV CRC who was receiving continuous 5-FU infusion and bolus 5-FU. The patient developed grade 2 PPE during the fourth cycle, which increased to grade 3 by the end of the sixth cycle despite the use of Udderly Smooth Balm® (Reddex Industries), a urea-based agent, and pyridoxine. The patient's treatment regimen was changed two additional times to reduce skin toxicity. A second case report documented PPE treatment of a patient with advanced pancreatic cancer who was receiving capecitabine 1,600 mg/m^2/day for six weeks, followed by maintenance 2,000 mg/m^2/day. PPE developed, and capecitabine was held, with improvement of PPE to grade 1 (Saif et al., 2007).

Use of emollients and moisturizers for EGFR inhibitor–induced rash: Only one case series was found that reported on the use of a topical urea-based emollient for EGFR inhibitor–induced rash. In this case series, 30 patients treated with cetuximab for CRC experienced acne-like rash—6 with grade 3, 18 with grade 2, and 6 with grade 1. All patients received topical 0.1% vitamin K_1 cream with urea beginning with the first noted rash. Improvement was noted in 8–18 days for all patients (Ocvirk & Rebersek, 2008).

Immune Modulator, Topical
One case report documented the use of topical pimecrolimus (Elidel®, Novartis Pharmaceuticals), an immune modulator, for the treatment of EGFR inhibitor–induced papulopustular cutaneous reaction accompanied by burning sensation on the face and pruritus on the scalp and upper body. The patient was given doxycycline 50 mg twice a day along with Elidel. This treatment was effective for this patient, as evidenced by a marked decrease in pruritus on the scalp and the burning sensation on the face (Lacouture, Boerner, & Lorusso, 2006).

Retinoids, Topical
Several authors reported results of studies and case reports related to the use of various retinoids for skin toxicity management. Results of the effectiveness of topical retinoids were mixed. One study was found in which topical tazarotene was used for EGFR inhibitor–associated rash (Scope et al., 2007). Two case series reported on the use of topical retinoids for management of rash, and one case was reported in which a topical retinoid was used for photosensitivity. Because of these combination treatments for rash, it is difficult to establish the effect of the individual components of the combined treatments in these studies, which limits the conclusions that can be drawn in relation to the effectiveness of retinoids in the treatment of skin toxicities.

Use of topical tazarotene: One randomized controlled trial (N = 48) studied the effectiveness of topical tazarotene 0.05% cream in resolving the EGFR inhibitor–induced rash. The cream was applied to just one side of the face with the rash for eight weeks. The results demonstrated no clinical benefit for the use of the tazarotene 0.05% cream. In fact, the cream was associated with significant irritation and was discontinued in one-third of the patients (Scope et al., 2007).

Use of topical retinoids in combination with other local and topical interventions: A case series described three case studies with the use of topical adapalene 0.1% gel in combination with other interventions for the treatment of EGFR inhibitor–induced rash. One patient used adapalene 0.1% gel nightly, along with benzoyl peroxide 4% gel applied in the morning, and had significant improvement in lesion count. Another patient had a reduction in lesion count using adapalene 0.1% gel applied twice daily, dilute acetic acid soaks, mupirocin cream three to four times daily, and minocycline 100 mg twice daily. The third patient applied topical adapalene 0.1% cream once daily, which resulted in partial improvement of the rash. Next, the patient was started on isotretinoin 20 mg once daily for one month, which was decreased to 20 mg every other day because of xerosis of the lips. This combination treatment caused dramatic clearing of the pustules (DeWitt et al., 2007).

Another case series described two patients who used tretinoin 0.025% cream twice a day, which led to improvement of the follicular lesions. One of these patients experienced aggravated scaling of the skin with this intervention (Van Doorn et al., 2002).

In addition, one case study discussed the use of a low-potency steroid, retinoid, and hydroquinone cream for drug-induced photosensitivity. This report showed no improvement in the area of photosensitivity (Kong, Fine, Stern, & Turner, 2009).

Steroids, Topical

Several case reports and the NCCN Task Force report discussed the use of topical steroids for skin toxicity (Burtness et al., 2009).

One report described a patient who was receiving cetuximab therapy and developed a follicular eruption on all cutaneous surfaces except the palmar, plantar, and mucosal surfaces. Kimyai-Asadi and Jih (2002) suggested treating the rash by combining therapies of topical corticosteroid (triamcinolone acetonide cream) and topical clindamycin and withholding the third dose of the cetuximab therapy. These interventions led to improvements in the eruptions in two weeks. When the cetuximab therapy was resumed, the skin eruptions worsened. This was partially controlled using topical steroids and anti-inflammatory medications (Kimyai-Asadi & Hih, 2002).

Jacot and colleagues (2004) described one patient with CRC who received cetuximab and developed a rash within three days. The authors suggested that the use of corticoid cream, together with erythromycin solution (4%), resulted in partial resolution of rash located on the trunk. This report did not record the time for resolution of the rash (Jacot et al., 2004).

The NCCN Task Force report suggested that topical steroids and antibiotics may be useful for treating skin rash associated with EGFR inhibitor therapy, but they noted that no data from randomized clinical trials exist to support this approach (Burtness et al., 2009).

In one case report, a combined treatment of a topical steroid, retinoid, and hydroquinone cream were used for treatment of a rash related to photosensitivity. No improvement was reported for the intervention (Kong et al., 2009).

SYSTEMIC INTERVENTIONS

A variety of systemic treatments to manage skin toxicities have been reported, including amifostine, systemic antibiotics, oral steroids, cyclooxygenase-2 (COX-2) inhibitors, pregabalin, pyridoxine, and vitamin E. Systemic antibiotics have been used frequently, and most reports of this intervention were found in patients receiving EGFR inhibitor therapy. Interpretation of the evidence related to the use of systemic antibiotics is complicated by the fact that in most reports, this intervention was usually accompanied by multiple other treatments. Tan and Chan's systematic review (2009) noted that the use of antibiotics may hold some promise but that high-quality evidence in this area is lacking. NCCN also noted that antibiotic use has been based upon clinical experience and expert preference rather than on strong research evidence (Burtness et al., 2009).

Amifostine Use for PPE

Two studies were found in which amifostine was used for PPE. Results suggested some effect; however, both studies involved very small sample sizes.

In an open-label study of patients with advanced cancer (N = 22), the incidence and severity of PPE were reduced with the addition of amifostine (500 mg/m^2 IV) to the PLD regimen (Lyass et al., 2000). In another phase II study of patients with multiple myeloma (N = 12) receiving PLD, vincristine, and dexamethasone, the results demonstrated that the addition of amifostine (200 mg/m^2 IV) appeared to ameliorate or prevent PPE symptoms (Jajeh, Agbernadzo, Zalzaleh, Koko, & Boek, 2002).

Antibiotics, Systemic

Seven references and one systematic review were found that reported on the use of systemic antibiotics for rash and paronychia in patients receiving EGFR inhibitor therapy. A report of two cases reviewed the use of IV minocycline for paronychia with positive culture for methicillin-resistant *Staphylococcus aureus* (MRSA). Two randomized controlled trials and one descriptive study were found that reported on the use of oral antibiotics in the tetracycline group for EGFR inhibitor–induced rash, and three case reports described the effects of oral antibiotics on paronychia. One case series report discussed the use of topical or oral antibiotics in combination with steroids (Fox, 2007).

Use of systemic antibiotics for EGFR inhibitor–induced rash: Two randomized, placebo-controlled clinical trials were conducted with study patients taking an EGFR inhibitor and initiating an oral antibiotic on day 1 of the EGFR inhibitor therapy. Both studies reported a less severe rash in the groups receiving the antibiotic than in the groups receiving a placebo. In one study conducted by Jatoi and colleagues (2008), patients with cancer (N = 61) received 500 mg of oral tetracycline twice daily for 28 days versus placebo. The antibiotic was started on day 1 of initiation of any EGFR inhibitor therapy. The tetracycline group (n = 31) reported less severe rash and better quality of life (Jatoi et al., 2008).

Scope and colleagues (2007) conducted another randomized, double-blind, placebo-controlled study with patients with CRC (N = 48) who were receiving cetuximab. The antibiotic, minocycline 100 mg a day, was started on day 1 of initiation of cetuximab therapy. Scope and colleagues (2007) reported that patients who received minocycline 100 mg a day (n = 24) had decreased severity of rash over those patients who received placebo (n = 24).

In a small open-label, descriptive study, 18 of 19 patients who were taking EGFR inhibitors developed a grade 2 rash and received doxycycline or minocycline 100 mg a day. More than 50% of these 18 patients had a complete response to oral antibiotic treatment. In addition, all patients were started on topical nadifloxacin or clindamycin, with or without benzoyl peroxide (de Noronha e Menezes et al., 2009).

Several case reports discussed the noted benefits of topical and oral antibiotics and rash reduction or disappearance. These include

1. DeWitt et al. (2007) reported on a patient who was taking an EGFR inhibitor and whose rash significantly improved on minocycline 100 mg twice a day with topical adapalene 0.1% gel.

2. Micantonio et al. (2005) reported decreasing rash severity in a second cycle and eliminating the recurrence of rash in a third cycle of a patient receiving an EGFR inhibitor plus chemotherapy by taking minocycline 200 mg daily for 7 days, then lymecycline 300 mg for the rest of cycles.

3. Lacouture et al. (2006) reported the benefit of doxycycline 50 mg twice daily with topical pimecrolimus in a patient taking an EGFR inhibitor. The researchers reported a decrease in rash, pruritus, and dryness. The patient's quality of life was also reported as improved.

4. Molinari et al. (2005) reported on 11 patients who received EGFR inhibitors and developed skin rash. At least five patients also reported pruritus. Two patients received doxycycline plus a local retinoid, one with doxycycline plus benzoyl peroxide and one with doxycycline alone. All patients showed improvement. No details regarding doses or routes of drugs or specific skin assessment findings were reported.

Two case studies reported on the combined approach of treating EGFR inhibitor–induced rash with oral antibiotics and suspension of EGFR inhibitor therapy. Robert, Soria, and Chosidow (2006) reported a case of a patient on an EGFR inhibitor who developed a rash and began taking doxycycline 200 mg for three weeks and noted improvement in the rash. The rash returned at week 11 and was cultured positive for *Staphylococcus aureus*. The EGFR inhibitor therapy was stopped for one week, and the antibiotic was restarted, with benefit (Robert et al., 2006). Vezzoli and colleagues (2008) also reported withholding treatment for rash incidence. Their patient was receiving EGFR inhibitor therapy and developed a rash. The patient was treated with clarithromycin 500 mg twice daily for seven days along with boric acid and zinc oxide. In addition, the EGFR inhibitor therapy was withheld for two weeks. The patient's rash disappeared, and EGFR inhibitor therapy was restarted. The rash reappeared, which caused a repeat of the scenario and intervention (Vezzoli et al., 2008).

Tan and Chan (2009) summarized findings from 2 randomized controlled trials, 3 case series and 10 case reports across a total of 156 patients. From their review, they recommended that systemic antibiotics, specifically minocycline or doxycycline, should be used to treat more severe rash. They noted that the review had a number of limitations given the type of evidence available and that well-designed studies with appropriate follow-up are needed for appropriate evaluation of therapeutic agents for this problem.

Use of systemic antibiotics for EGFR inhibitor–induced paronychia: Several researchers reported various systemic antibiotic therapies used for EGFR inhibitor–induced paronychia and their effectiveness. Fox (2007) reviewed many of these case reports of patients experiencing EGFR inhibitor–induced paronychia.

Dainichi and colleagues (2003) discussed two case reports of patients receiving gefitinib, a tyrosine kinase inhibitor of EGFR. They noted that both patients experienced eruption of paronychia with painful granulomatous papules, which cultured positive for MRSA. IV minocycline was administered for seven days, with ongoing topical treatment of dressing and betamethasone, with a decrease in the size of papules over a few weeks (Dainichi, Tanaka, Tsuruta, Furue, & Noda, 2003).

Nakano and Nakamura (2003) reported three cases of patients who received gefitinib and experienced paronychia. They were treated with topical and systemic antibiotic therapies, which were not effective.

Chang et al. (2004) reported two case studies of patients who were receiving gefitinib. Both patients experienced paronychia and were treated with minocycline and gefitinib dose interruption. One patient had a positive culture for *Staphylococcus aureus*. Paronychia symptoms were improved for both patients, but these symptoms waxed and waned with return of gefitinib therapy.

Suh et al. (2006) reported on one female patient with CRC who was receiving cetuximab, an EGFR inhibitor. She developed paronychia and was treated with topical mupirocin twice daily and cephalexin 500 mg four times a day without improvement. Treatment with cetuximab was also stopped. Doxycycline 100 mg twice a day was then initiated and resulted in an improvement of the patient's ability to perform daily living activities.

Cyclooxygenase-2 (COX-2) Inhibitors

In a retrospective study of patients with CRC (N = 67) who were receiving capecitabine, the addition of a COX-2 inhibitor (200 mg twice daily) resulted in the reduction of grade 1 PPE (p = 0.037) and of grade 2 PPE (p = 0.11) (Lin et al., 2002).

Pregabalin

In one case report of a 62-year-old man with locally advanced adenocarcinoma of the nasal cavity who was receiving treatment with cetuximab, the authors reported development of grade 3 skin toxicity on the scalp, face, and thorax with intense pruritus. The patient had distress related to sleep deprivation, depression, anxiety, and asthenia. Symptoms were unrelieved by oral promethazine 50 mg and topical anti-inflammatory cream. The patient was given pregabalin 75 mg orally twice daily, which was titrated to 100 mg twice daily. This treatment resulted in a decrease in all cutaneous symptoms. He continued on pregabalin for the duration of therapy (Porzio et al., 2006).

Systemic Steroids for PPE and Rash

Three small studies (Drake et al., 2004; Kollmannsberger et al., 2000; Mangili et al., 2008) and one case report (Titgan, 1997) were found that discussed the use of systemic steroids for the prevention and management of PPE. Another single case was reported in which premedication with oral dexamethasone was used to prevent rash associated with gemcitabine (Kanai et al., 2010).

The evidence for the effectiveness of oral and topical steroids in preventing or treating PPE is mixed. Although case studies of pretreatment steroids to prevent PPE associated with chemotherapy have reported positive results, very few cases have been reported, and no randomized studies were found. Overall, it is difficult to ascertain the direct effect of systemic steroids because they may be part of numerous premedication regimens (e.g., antiemetic and dexamethasone). Study samples reported were also extremely small.

Use of systemic steroids for PPE: Drake et al. (2004) conducted a study of women with gynecologic cancers (N = 23) who were receiving PLD (50 mg/m^2 on a 28-day cycle). They found that oral dexamethasone was effective in preventing or resolving PLD-induced PPE symptoms. Nine patients developed PPE. Six of the nine patients received oral dexamethasone and had complete or near complete resolution of the PPE. Three of the nine patients did not receive the dexamethasone and required treatment delays and dose reduction.

Kollmannsberger et al. (2006) conducted a study of patients receiving PLD (N = 19). PLD doses varied from 40 mg/m^2 to 60 mg/m^2, and frequency varied from 14- to 28-day cycles. They found that the incidence of PPE caused by PLD appeared to decrease with concomitant dexamethasone (8 mg, by mouth, twice daily, from day 1 until day +5 of each cycle) and pyridoxine (100 mg orally, twice daily, continuously).

Mangili et al. (2008) conducted a study of the effectiveness of PPE prevention strategies for patients receiving PLD (N = 25). When a multivariate analysis was performed, they determined that the use of steroid prophylaxis (dexamethasone 8 mg by mouth, taken 12 hours before PLD infusion) was not a significant factor in the prevention of PPE because nine of the patients developed PPE.

Titgan (1997) reported on a case study of a 64-year-old patient with stage IV ovarian cancer who was being treated with PLD (50 mg/m^2 every four weeks). The patient was premedicated with a variety of premedication, including dexamethasone 20 mg IV, on the day of treatment. After the third cycle of chemotherapy, she developed an erythematous maculopapular rash. She was then instructed to take dexamethasone 8 mg orally twice daily, starting 24 hours before treatment and continuing for 5 days at the same dose and tapered over the next 48 hours. This regimen was successful in preventing the dermatologic reactions of PLD (Titgan, 1997).

Use of systemic steroids for gemcitabine-induced rash: Kanai et al. (2010) also reported a case series of patients who received gemcitabine (N = 107). Four of these patients developed an extensive skin rash. Pretreatment with 4–8 mg IV dexamethasone was not sufficient to prevent gemcitabine-induced skin rash. However, when they premedicated the patients (n = 4) with 20 mg dexamethasone prior to treatment in order to prevent rash, the patients did not develop a rash after being rechallenged with gemcitabine.

Vitamin B$_6$ (Pyridoxine), Oral
In several studies, the results demonstrated that the use of oral pyridoxine may reduce the incidence and/or severity of PPE symptoms associated with specific drug administration (continuous infusion 5-FU, PLD). The oral vitamin B$_6$ (average dosages ranging from 50–300 mg/day) was used either alone or in combination with other preventive interventions (i.e., oral steroids, strategies to reduce heat and friction to skin, emollients) (Eng et al., 2001; Fabian et al., 1990; Gordon et al., 1995; Jajeh et al., 2002; Mangili et al., 2008; Saif et al., 2007; Vukelja, Baker, Burris, Keeling, & Von Hoff, 1993).

The effectiveness of pyridoxine itself cannot be adequately determined because reported treatments with pyridoxine are combined with multiple other interventions. Results from one large retrospective chart review (N = 198) found that the use of pyridoxine to prevent PPE symptoms was not supported; however, the use of pyridoxine to manage PPE symptoms was favorable (p < 0.001) (Mortimer et al., 2003).

Vitamin E, Oral
Five cases of patients with breast cancer who were receiving docetaxel and capecitabine treatment and developed PPE symptoms were reported. The results remonstrated that oral vitamin E (300 mg) was effective in resolving PPE symptoms (Kara, Sahin, & Erkisi, 2006).

OTHER INTERVENTIONS

Electrodessication
In a case study of one patient with non-small cell lung cancer who was receiving gefitinib, paronychia developed on day 20. This was successfully treated with electrodessication of the larger lesions (Dainichi et al., 2003).

Minimizing Sun Exposure
The EGFR in keratinocytes can be directly affected by ultraviolet-B light irradiation (Hussein, 2005); therefore, most experts recommend avoidance of sun exposure for patients who are receiving EGFR inhibitor agents. Two case studies were found specifically noting minimizing sun exposure to manage skin photosensitivity secondary to vandetanib therapy. In both cases, pigmentation changes were noted to improve with sun avoidance and worsen with exposure (Chang, Chang, Hui, & Yang, 2009; Kong et al., 2009).

Nicotine Patch
In a case study of one patient with CRC who was receiving 24-hour 5-FU infusions, a nicotine patch (7 mg) was applied to the patient's skin during the infusion and was found to be effective for dermatitis (Kingsley, 1994).

Effectiveness Unlikely

Interventions for which lack of effectiveness has been demonstrated by negative evidence from well-designed controlled trials using small samples or guidelines developed from evidence and supported by expert opinion

There are no interventions as of February 2010.

Not Recommended for Practice

Interventions for which lack of effectiveness or harmfulness has been demonstrated by strong evidence from rigorously conducted studies, meta-analyses, or systematic reviews, or interventions where the costs, burden, or harms associated with the intervention exceed anticipated benefit

There are no interventions as of February 2010.

Expert Opinion

Low-risk interventions that are (1) consistent with sound clinical practice, (2) suggested by an expert in a peer-reviewed publication (journal or book chapter), and (3) for which limited evidence exists. An expert is an individual with peer-reviewed journal publications in the domain of interest.

Although controlled studies to assess the individual contribution of the following interventions are lacking, experts appear to agree on a number of recommendations related to the care of patients experiencing skin reactions to cancer treatments. Many of these recommendations were also employed concurrently with the interventions noted in other evidence described in this resource.

AVOIDING TISSUE PRESSURE, IRRITATION, AND TRAUMA

Several measures are recommended to prevent and minimize the extent and discomfort of PPE and to prevent paronychia formation. These measures include (a) avoiding prolonged friction or pressure and (b) avoiding extreme temperature exposures or irritation to the skin, especially the hands and feet and including the nail beds (Edwards, 2003; Galimont-Collen, Vos, Lavrijsen, Ouwerkerk, & Gelderblom, 2007; Jatoi et al., 2008; Krozely, 2004; Moore, 2007; Scheithauer & Blum, 2004; Segaert & Van Cutsem, 2005; Sipples, 2006; Swenson & Bell, 2010; Webster-Gandy, How, & Harrold, 2007).

APPLICATION OF WARM OR COOL SOAKS

Warm water soaks of the fingers and toes may provide comfort and prevent paronychial infection (Viale, 2006). Cool soaks or cool pack applications have been described as helpful to provide relief for PPE and pruritus symptoms (Agero et al., 2006; Edwards, 2003; Frye, 2009; Jatoi et al., 2008; Lacouture, Reilly, Gerami, & Guitart, 2008; Segaert et al., 2005; Shah et al., 2005).

ANTIHISTAMINES

A number of experts recommend the use of topical or systemic antihistamines to manage pruritus associated with rash lesions, photosensitivity reactions, or xerosis (Agero et al., 2006; Eaby, Culkin, & Lacouture, 2008; Herbst, LoRusso, Purdom, & Ward, 2003; Lacouture, 2007; Lacouture, Cotliar, & Mitchell, 2007; Lacouture et al., 2008, Perez-Soler et al., 2005).

DERMATOLOGY CONSULT

For patients with blistering and ulceration, topical wound care and dermatology consult is recommended (Gerbrecht, 2003).

LOTIONS AND MOISTURIZERS

Experts recommend regularly and gently applying moisturizing creams or topical emollients to prevent PPE or at the appearance of grade 1 PPE symptoms. Patients should apply at night and wear loose-fitting cotton gloves or socks (Burtness et al., 2009; Dunsford, 2008; Eaby et al., 2008; Edwards, 2003; Gerbrecht, 2003; Saif et al., 2007; Wilkes & Doyle, 2005).

PATIENT EDUCATION

For preventing and minimizing PPE, patient education is a key intervention. This includes teaching patients to (a) assess pressure-sensitive areas, (b) report signs and symptoms of PPE as soon as possible, and (c) use restorative and prophylactic strategies to minimize the likelihood or degree that PPE may develop (Wilkes & Doyle, 2005).

TOPICAL ANESTHETICS

For severe pruritus, use of a topical numbing agent such as pramoxine or lidocaine may offer relief (Eaby et al., 2008; Lacouture, 2007; Lacouture et al., 2007).

TECHNIQUES TO PREVENT AND MANAGE PARONYCHIA

Regular use of a topical paste consisting of an antiseptic, such as chlorhexidine, and an anti-yeast agent, such as nystatin, with the addition of a corticosteroid in the development of a severe lesion was reported as helpful (Segaert & Van Cutsem, 2005). Paronychial lesions associated with EGFR inhibitors are generally of an inflammatory, not infectious, origin. Because secondary infections can establish easily, culturing of persistent or pustular lesions is recommended (Burtness et al., 2009; Lacouture et al., 2007; Segaert & Van Cutsem, 2005). Topical agents, such as silver nitrate, ferric subsulfate solution, and aluminum acetate (Burrow's solution), and cellulose sponges to pack affected areas, can be used (Burtness et al., 2009). NCCN has also suggested the use of 4% thymol in alcohol or bleach soaks to prevent infection and use of topical corticosteroid cream for inflammatory, noninfected paronychia. In addition, patients with paronychia should not use isotretinoin (Burtness et al., 2009).

TECHNIQUES TO PREVENT AND MANAGE XEROSIS AND PRURITUS

Interventions include suggesting that patients avoid overheating by wearing loose-fitting, light cotton fabrics and maintaining adequate fluid intake (Pyle et al., 2008) and use of ammonium lactate 12% lotion (Lacouture et al., 2007). Use of medical-grade cyanoacrylate (also known as 2-octyl cyanoacrylate and DermaBond® [Johnson & Johnson]) has been noted to be of use in closing fissures secondary to xerosis (Esper, Gale, & Muehlbauer, 2007; Segaert & Van Cutsem, 2005).

DOSE MODIFICATION

The most effective management for several significant skin reactions (e.g., grades 2–4 EGFR inhibitor–induced rash, PPE, or other skin reactions) is treatment interruption, dose reduction or delay, or lengthening the interval between drug administrations. These interventions normally lead to a rapid subsidence of symptoms (Gordon et al., 1995; Janusch et al., 2006; Jatoi, Green, Rowland, Sargent, & Alberts, 2009; Lassere & Hoff, 2004; Lorusso et al., 2007; Lynch et al., 2007; Markman et al., 2000; O'Shaughnessy et al., 2001; Perez-Soler et al., 2005; Rose et al., 2001).

A note of caution regarding dosage modification: because of the association between cutaneous side effects and the potential for response and survival benefit, many authors suggest maintaining treatment dosing regimens when at all possible (Burtness et al., 2009; Lacouture et al., 2008; Lynch et al., 2007; Perez-Soler et al., 2004; Wagner & Lacouture, 2007).

Areas for Research

Three areas of future research are vital to improving evidence-based care for patients experiencing cutaneous reactions to cancer therapies:

1. Development and validation of instruments to measure clinician and patient evaluation of the extent, severity, and functional interference of cutaneous reactions. Valid and reliable measurement of toxicities and symptoms is necessary in order to describe and assess the effectiveness of treatments. The current methods of clinician measurement of skin toxicities are not specific for the diverse cutaneous reactions seen with newer cancer therapies. Clinicians report that the current measurements are inadequate to effectively describe the extent and severity of these reactions. Valid clinician rating scales measuring the extent and severity of different cutaneous reactions with established inter-rater reliability are needed. Valid patient-reported outcome (PRO) measures of the effect of skin diseases on patients' quality of life exist. However, these measures do not have proven validity and reliability for the cutaneous reactions to cancer therapies. Because they were designed to measure skin diseases, they may not be completely valid for cutaneous reactions. Testing of these current PRO instruments for validity and reliability in patients with different cutaneous reactions, as well as development of PRO instruments specific for cutaneous reactions, is needed. Concurrent validity with functional status is especially critical for both clinician and PRO measurements.

2. Descriptive studies to delineate the types, incidence, and severity of cutaneous reactions and their effect on patient functioning. Studies describing the occurrence, incidence, severity, and natural course of these skin reactions are necessary. Although some descriptions of these reactions exist, very few studies have systematically measured and reported the occurrence and severity of these reactions with different therapies over time. The simultaneous occurrence of multiple cutaneous toxicities and the concurrence of other symptoms also have not been described. Because some of these cutaneous reactions are reported to improve with time, it is especially important to understand the natural course of these skin reactions if interventions to relieve them are to be tested.

3. Randomized controlled trials to test the efficacy of interventions compared to placebos and to each other in preventing cutaneous reactions, decreasing severity, and maintaining patient function. The current available evidence is insufficient regarding interventions for

cancer treatment–related cutaneous reactions. However, many interventions have been reported in case studies, case series, and studies with smaller sample sizes or are recommended by experts. Some studies have reported the effectiveness of multiple interventions used in combination, which increases the difficulty in determining the effectiveness of one specific intervention. Randomized controlled trials testing these interventions against placebos and against each other are needed to provide evidence for the true efficacy of these interventions.

Search Strategy

Computerized literature searching was done using the consolidated PICO terms as outlined below. No date range restriction was employed, and additional manual retrieval was done for key findings from the literature. The limitations of adults and English language were used. The final literature search was performed in February 2010.

Patient/Problem: Patients with cancer who are receiving chemotherapy, biotherapy, targeted therapy, or any type of cancer treatment and who experience skin reactions, skin toxicities, macular rash, papular rash, maculopapular rash, follicular rash, paronychia, nail changes, nail inflammation, acneform rash, pruritus, itch, xerosis, dry skin, palmar-plantar erythrodysesthesia, hand-foot syndrome, photosensitivity

Intervention: None specified

Comparison: Standard care

Outcome: Improvement in or prevention of skin reactions

Type of Question: Prevention or treatment

Databases Used: PubMed, CINAHL®, EMBASE®, Cochrane Collaboration, Google™ Scholar.

Inclusion Criteria: Patients with cancer, receiving cancer treatment, English language

Exclusion Criteria: Patients receiving radiation therapy or combined radiation and chemotherapy

Definitions of the interventions are available at **www.ons.org/research/PEP**. Literature search completed through February 2010.

References

Adams, D.H., & Nutt, T. (2006). A case report and discussion of cetuximab-induced folliculitis. *American Journal of Clinical Dermatology, 7*, 333–336.

Agero, A.L.C., Dusza, S.W., Benvenuto-Andrade, C., Busam, K.J., Myskowski, P., & Halpern, A.C. (2006). Dermatologic side effects associated with the epidermal growth factor receptor inhibitors. *Journal of the American Academy of Dermatology, 55*, 657–670. doi:10.1016/j.jaad.2005.10.010

Alexandrescu, D.T., Vaillant, J.G., & Dasanu, C.A. (2007). Effect of treatment with a colloidal oatmeal lotion on the acneform eruption induced by epidermal growth factor receptor and multiple tyrosine-kinase inhibitors. *Clinical and Experimental Dermatology, 32*, 71–74. doi:10.1111/j.1365-2230.2006.02285.x

Boucher, K.W., Davidson, K., Mirakhur, B., Goldberg, J., & Heymann, W.R. (2002). Paronychia induced by cetuximab, an antiepidermal growth factor receptor antibody. *Journal of the American Academy of Dermatology, 47*, 632–633.

Burtness, B., Anadkat, M., Basti, S., Hughes, M., Lacouture, M.E., McClure, J.S., ... Spencer, S. (2009). NCCN Task Force report: Management of dermatologic and other toxicities associated with EGFR inhibition in patients with cancer. *Journal of the National Comprehensive Cancer Network, 7*(Suppl. 1), S5–S21.

Chang, C.H., Chang, J.W., Hui, C.Y., & Yang, C.H. (2009). Severe photosensitivity reaction to vandetanib. *Journal of Clinical Oncology, 27*, e114–e115. doi:10.1200/JCO.2009.21.8479

Chang, G.C., Yang, T.Y., Chen, K.C., Yin, M.C., Wang, R.C., & Lin, Y.C. (2004). Complications of therapy in cancer patients: Case 1. Paronychia and skin hyperpigmentation induced by gefitinib in advanced non-small-cell lung cancer. *Journal of Clinical Oncology, 22*, 4646–4648. doi:10.1200/JCO.2004.02.168

Chin, S.F., Tchen, N., Oza, A.M., Moore, M.J., Warr, D., & Siu, L.L. (2001). Use of Bag Balm as topical treatment of palmar-plantar erythrodysesthesia syndrome (PPES) in patients receiving selected chemotherapy agents [Abstract 1632]. *Proceedings of the American Society of Clinical Oncology, 20,* 409a.

Dainichi, T., Tanaka, M., Tsuruta, N., Furue, M., & Noda, K. (2003). Development of multiple paronychia and periungual granulation in patients treated with gefitinib, an inhibitor of epidermal growth factor receptor. *Dermatology, 207,* 324–325. doi:10.1159/000073100

de Noronha e Menezes, N.M., Lima, R., Moreira, A., Varela, P., Barroso, A., Baptista, A., & Parente, B. (2009). Description and management of cutaneous side effects during erlotinib and cetuximab treatment in lung and colorectal cancer patients: A prospective and descriptive study of 19 patients. *European Journal of Dermatology, 19,* 248–251. doi:10.1684/ejd.2009.0650

DeWitt, C.A., Siroy, A.E., & Stone, S.P. (2007). Acneiform eruptions associated with epidermal growth factor–targeted chemotherapy. *Journal of the American Academy of Dermatology, 56,* 500–505. doi:10.1016/j.jaad.2006.06.046

Drake, R.D., Lin, W.M., King, M., Farrar, D., Miller, D.S., & Coleman, R.L. (2004). Oral dexamethasone attenuates Doxil-induced palmar-plantar erythrodysesthesias in patients with recurrent gynecologic malignancies. *Gynecologic Oncology, 94,* 320–324. doi:10.1016/j.ygyno.2004.05.027

Dunsford, J. (2008). Nursing management of epidermal growth factor receptor inhibitor-induced toxicities. *Clinical Journal of Oncology Nursing, 12,* 405–407. doi:10.1188/08.CJON.405-407

Eaby, B., Culkin, A., & Lacouture, M.E. (2008). An interdisciplinary consensus on managing skin reactions associated with human epidermal growth factor receptor inhibitors. *Clinical Journal of Oncology Nursing, 12,* 283–290. doi:10.1188/08.CJON.283-290

Edwards, S.J. (2003). Prevention and treatment of adverse effects related to chemotherapy for recurrent ovarian cancer. *Seminars in Oncology Nursing, 19*(3, Suppl. 1), 19–39.

Eng, C., Mauer, A.M., Fleming, G.F., Bertucci, D., Rotmensch, J., Jacobs, R.H., & Ratain, M.J. (2001). Phase I study of pegylated liposomal doxorubicin, paclitaxel, and cisplatin in patients with advanced solid tumors. *Annals of Oncology, 12,* 1743–1747. Retrieved from http://annonc.oxfordjournals.org/content/12/12/1743.long

Esper, P., Gale, D., & Muehlbauer, P. (2007). What kind of rash is it?: Deciphering the dermatologic toxicities of biologic and targeted therapies. *Clinical Journal of Oncology Nursing, 11,* 659–666. doi:10.1188/07.CJON.659-666

Fabian, C.J., Molina, R., Slavik, M., Dahlberg, S., Giri, S., & Stephens, R. (1990). Pyridoxine therapy for palmar-plantar erythrodysesthesia associated with continuous 5-fluorouracil infusion. *Investigational New Drugs, 8,* 57–63.

Fluhr, J.W., Miteva, M., Primavera, G., Ziemer, M., Elsner, P., & Berardesca, E. (2007). Functional assessment of a skin care system in patients on chemotherapy. *Skin Pharmacology and Physiology, 20,* 253–259. doi:10.1159/000104423

Fox, L.P. (2007). Nail toxicity associated with epidermal growth factor receptor inhibitor therapy. *Journal of the American Academy of Dermatology, 56,* 460–465. doi:10.1016/j.jaad.2006.09.013

Frye, D.K. (2009). Capecitabine-based combination therapy for breast cancer: Implications for nurses. *Oncology Nursing Forum, 36,* 105–113. doi:10.1188/09.ONF.105-113

Galimont-Collen, A.F., Vos, L.E., Lavrijsen, A.P., Ouwerkerk, J., & Gelderblom, H. (2007). Classification and management of skin, hair, nail and mucosal side-effects of epidermal growth factor receptor (EGFR) inhibitors. *European Journal of Cancer, 43,* 845–851. doi:10.1016/j.ejca.2006.11.016

Gerbrecht, B.M. (2003). Current Canadian experience with capecitabine: Partnering with patients to optimize therapy. *Cancer Nursing, 26,* 161–167.

Gordon, K.B., Tajuddin, A., Guitart, J., Kuzel, T.M., Eramo, L.R., & Von Roenn, J. (1995). Hand-foot syndrome associated with liposome-encapsulated doxorubicin therapy. *Cancer, 75,* 2169–2173. doi:10.1002/1097-0142(19950415)75:8<2169::AID-CNCR2820750822>3.0.CO;2-H

Gutzmer, R., Werfel, T., Mao, R., Kapp, A., & Elsner, J. (2005). Successful treatment with oral isotretinoin of acneiform skin lesions associated with cetuximab therapy. *British Journal of Dermatology, 153,* 842–868. doi:10.1111/j.1365-2133.2005.06835.x

Herbst, R.S., LoRusso, P.M., Purdom, M., & Ward, D. (2003). Dermatologic side effects associated with gefitinib therapy: Clinical experience and management. *Clinical Lung Cancer, 4,* 366–369. doi:10.3816/CLC.2003.n.016

Hussein, M.R. (2005). Ultraviolet radiation and skin cancer: Molecular mechanisms. *Journal of Cutaneous Pathology, 32,* 191–205. doi:10.1111/j.0303-6987.2005.00281.x

Jacot, W., Bessis, D., Jorda, E., Ychou, M., Fabbro, M., Pujol, J.L., & Guillot, B. (2004). Acneiform eruption induced by epidermal growth factor receptor inhibitors in patients with solid tumours. *British Journal of Dermatology, 151,* 238–241. doi:10.1111/j.1365-2133.2004.06026.x

Jajeh, A., Agbernadzo, B., Zalzaleh, G., Koko, I., & Boek, M. (2002). Aminofostine in the prevention of liposomal doxorubicin induced palmar-plantar erythrodysesthesia (PPE) [Abstract 5115]. *Blood, 11,* 388b.

Janusch, M., Fischer, M., Marsch, W., Holzhausen, H.J., Kegel, T., & Helmbold, P. (2006). The hand-foot syndrome—A frequent secondary manifestation in antineoplastic chemotherapy. *European Journal of Dermatology, 16,* 494–499.

Jatoi, A., Green, E.M., Rowland, K.M., Jr., Sargent, D.J., & Alberts, S.R. (2009). Clinical predictors of severe cetuximab-induced rash: Observations from 933 patients enrolled in North Central Cancer Treatment Group Study N0147. *Oncology, 77,* 120–123. doi:10.1159/000229751

Jatoi, A., Rowland, K., Sloan, J.A., Gross, H.M., Fishkin, P.A., Kahanic, S.P., ... Loprinzi, C.L. (2008). Tetracycline to prevent epidermal growth factor receptor inhibitor-induced skin rashes: Results of a placebo-controlled trial from the North Central Cancer Treatment Group (N03CB). *Cancer, 113,* 847–853. doi:10.1002/cncr.23621

Kanai, M., Matsumoto, S., Nishimura, T., Matsumura, Y., Hatano, E., Mori, A., ... Chiba, T. (2010). Premedication with 20 mg dexamethasone effectively prevents relapse of extensive skin rash associated with gemcitabine monotherapy. *Annals of Oncology, 21,* 189–190. doi:10.1093/annonc/mdp513

Kara, I.O., Sahin, B., & Erkisi, M. (2006). Palmar-plantar erythrodysesthesia due to docetaxel-capecitabine therapy is treated with vitamin E without dose reduction. *Breast, 15,* 413–423. doi:10.1016/j.breast.2005.07.007

Kimyai-Asadi, A., & Jih, M.H. (2002). Follicular toxic effects of chimeric anti-epidermal growth factor receptor antibody cetuximab used to treat human solid tumors. *Archives of Dermatology, 138,* 129–131. doi:10.1001/archderm.138.1.129

Kingsley, E.C. (1994). 5-fluorouracil dermatitis prophylaxis with a nicotine patch [Letter]. *Annals of Internal Medicine, 120,* 813.

Kollmannsberger, C., Mayer, F., Harstrick, A., Honecker, F., Vanhofer, U., Oberhoff, C., ... Bokemeyer, C. (2000). Reduction of skin toxicity of pegylated liposomal doxorubicin (PLD) by concomitant administration of dexamethasone and pyridoxine in patients (pts) with anthracycline-sensitive malignancies—A phase I/II trial [Abstract 623P]. *Annals of Oncology, 11*(Suppl. 4), 136. doi:10.1093/annonc/11.suppl_4.132

Kong, H.H., Fine, H.A., Stern, J.B., & Turner, M.L. (2009). Cutaneous pigmentation after photosensitivity induced by vandetanib therapy. *Archives of Dermatology, 145,* 923–925. doi:10.1001/archdermatol.2009.177

Krozely, P. (2004). Epidermal growth factor receptor tyrosine kinase inhibitors: Evolving role in the treatment of solid tumors. *Clinical Journal of Oncology Nursing, 8,* 163–168. doi:10.1188/04.CJON.163-168

Lacouture, M.E. (2007). Insights into the pathophysiology and management of dermatologic toxicities to EGFR-targeted therapies in colorectal cancer. *Cancer Nursing, 30*(4, Suppl. 1), S17–S26. doi:10.1097/01.NCC.0000281758.85704.9b

Lacouture, M.E., Boerner, S.A., & Lorusso, P.M. (2006). Non-rash skin toxicities associated with novel targeted therapies. *Clinical Lung Cancer, 8*(Suppl. 1), S36–S42.

Lacouture, M.E., Cotliar, J., & Mitchell, E.P. (2007). Clinical management of EGFRI dermatologic toxicities: US perspective. *Oncology, 21*(11, Suppl. 5), 17–21.

Lacouture, M.E., Maitland, M.L., Segaert, S., Setser, A., Baran, R., Fox, L.P., ... Trotti, A. (2010). A proposed EGFR inhibitor dermatologic adverse event-specific grading scale from the MASCC Skin Toxicity Study Group. *Supportive Care in Cancer, 18,* 509–522. doi:10.1007/s00520-009-0744-x

Lacouture, M.E., Reilly, L.M., Gerami, P., & Guitart, J. (2008). Hand foot skin reaction in cancer patients treated with the multikinase inhibitors sorafenib and sunitinib. *Annals of Oncology, 19,* 1955–1961. doi:10.1093/annonc/mdn389

Lassere, Y., & Hoff, P. (2004). Management of hand-foot syndrome in patients treated with capecitabine (Xeloda). *European Journal of Oncology Nursing, 8*(Suppl. 1), S31–S40. doi:10.1016/j.ejon.2004.06.007

Lee, M.W., Seo, C.W., Kim, S.W., Yang, H.J., Lee, H.W., Choi, J.H., ... Koh, J.K. (2004). Cutaneous side effects in non-small cell lung cancer patients treated with Iressa (ZD 1839), an inhibitor of epidermal growth factor. *Acta Dermato-Venereologica, 84,* 23–26.

Lin, E.H., Morris, J., Chau, N.K., Crane, C., Wolff, R., Janjan, N., ... Abbruzzese, J.L. (2002). Celecoxib attenuated capecitabine induced hand-and-foot syndrome (HFS) and diarrhea and improved time to tumor progression in metastatic colorectal cancer (MCRC) [Abstract 2364]. *Proceedings of the American Society of Clinical Oncology, 21*(Suppl.). Retrieved from http://www.asco.org/ASCOv2/Meetings/Abstracts?&vmview=abst_detail_view&confID=16&abstractID=2364

Lopez, A.M., Wallace, L., Dorr, R.T., Koff, M., Hersh, E.M., & Alberts, D.S. (1999). Topical DMSO treatment for pegylated liposomal doxorubicin-induced palmar-plantar erythrodysesthesia. *Cancer Chemotherapy and Pharmacology, 44,* 303–306. doi:10.1007/s002800050981

Lorusso, D., Di Stefano, A., Carone, V., Fagotti, A., Pisconti, S., & Scambia, G. (2007). Pegylated liposomal doxorubicin-related palmar-plantar erythrodysesthesia (hand-foot syndrome). *Annals of Oncology, 18,* 1159–1164. doi:10.1093/annonc/mdl477

Lyass, O., Uziely, B., Ben-Yosef, R., Tzemach, D., Heshing, N.I., Lotem, M., ... Gabizon, A. (2000). Correlation of toxicity with pharmacokinetics of pegylated liposomal doxorubicin (Doxil) in metastatic breast carcinoma. *Cancer, 89,* 1037–1047. doi:10.1002/1097-0142(20000901)89:5<1037::AID-CNCR13>3.0.CO;2-Z

Lynch, T.J., Jr., Kim, E.S., Eaby, B., Garey, J., West, D.P., & Lacouture, M.E. (2007). Epidermal growth factor receptor inhibitor-associated cutaneous toxicities: An evolving paradigm in clinical management. *Oncologist, 12,* 610–621. doi:10.1634/theoncologist.12-5-610

Mangili, G., Gentile, C., Rabaiotti, E., Pella, F., Petrone, M., Zanetto, F., & Ferrari, A. (2006). The role of regional cooling on prevention of palmar-plantar erythrodysesthesia in patients treated with pegylated liposomal doxorubicin [Abstract 677]. *International Journal of Gynecological Cancer, 16,* 790.

Mangili, G., Petrone, M., Gentile, C., De Marzi, P., Viganò, R., & Rabaiotti, E. (2008). Prevention strategies in palmar-plantar erythrodysesthesia onset: The role of regional cooling. *Gynecologic Oncology, 108,* 332–335. doi:10.1016/j.ygyno.2007.10.021

Markman, M., Kennedy, A., Webster, K., Peterson, G., Kulp, B., & Belinson, J. (2000). Phase 2 trial of liposomal doxorubicin (40 mg/m^2) in platinum/paclitaxel-refractory ovarian and fallopian tube cancers and primary carcinoma of the peritoneum. *Gynecologic Oncology, 78*(3, Pt. 1), 369–372. doi:10.1006/gyno.2000.5921

Micantonio, T., Fargnoli, M.C., Ricevuto, E., Ficorella, C., Marchetti, P., & Peris, K. (2005). Efficacy of treatment with tetracyclines to prevent acneiform eruption secondary to cetuximab therapy. *Archives of Dermatology, 141,* 1173–1174. doi:10.1001/archderm.141.9.1173

Molinari, E., De Quatrebarbes, J., André, T., & Aractingi, S. (2005). Cetuximab-induced acne. *Dermatology, 211,* 330–333. doi:10.1159/000088502

Molpus, K.L., Anderson, L.B., Craig, C.L., & Pulee, J.G. (2004). The effect of regional cooling on toxicity associated with intravenous infusion of pegylated liposomal doxorubicin in recurrent ovarian carcinoma. *Gynecologic Oncology, 93,* 513–516.

Moore, S. (2007). Managing treatment side effects in advanced breast cancer. *Seminars in Oncology Nursing, 23*(4, Suppl. 2), S23–S30. doi:10.1016/j.soncn.2007.10.005

Mortimer, J.E., Lauman, M.K., Tan, B., Dempsey, C.L., Shillington, A.C., & Hutchins, K.S. (2003). Pyridoxine treatment and prevention of hand-and-foot syndrome in patients receiving capecitabine. *Journal of Oncology Pharmacy Practice, 9,* 161–166. doi:10.1191/1078155203jp116oa

Nakano, J., & Nakamura, M. (2003). Paronychia induced by gefitinib, an epidermal growth factor receptor tyrosine kinase inhibitor. *Journal of Dermatology, 30,* 261–262.

Ocvirk, J., & Cencelj, S. (2009). Management of cutaneous side-effects of cetuximab therapy in patients with metastatic colorectal cancer. *Journal of the European Academy of Dermatology and Venereology, 24,* 453–459. doi:10.1111/j.1468-3083.2009.03446.x

Ocvirk, J., & Rebersek, M. (2008). Managing cutaneous side effects with K1 vitamine creme reduces cutaneous toxicities induced by cetuximab. *Journal of Clinical Oncology, 26*(Suppl. 15), Abstract 20750.

O'Shaughnessy, J. A., Blum, J., Moiseyenko, V., Jones, S.E., Miles, D., Bell, D., ... Laws, S. (2001). Randomized, open-label, phase II trial of oral capecitabine (Xeloda) vs. a reference arm of intravenous CMF (cyclophosphamide, methotrexate and 5-fluorouracil) as first-line therapy for advanced/metastatic breast cancer. *Annals of Oncology, 12,* 1247–1254. Retrieved from http://annonc.oxfordjournals.org/content/12/9/1247.long

Pendharkar, D., & Goyal, H. (2004). Novel and effective management of capecitabine induced hand foot syndrome. *Journal of Clinical Oncology, 22*(Suppl. 14), Abstract 8105. Retrieved from http://www.asco.org/ASCOv2/Meetings/Abstracts?&vmview=abst_detail_view&confID=26&abstractID=3308

Perez-Soler, R., Chachoua, A., Hammond, L.A., Rowinsky, E.K., Huberman, M., Karp, D., ... Bonomi, P. (2004). Determinants of tumor response and survival with erlotinib in patients with non-small cell lung cancer. *Journal of Clinical Oncology, 22,* 3238–3247. doi:10.1200/JCO.2004.11.057

Perez-Soler, R., Delord, J.P., Halpern, A., Kelly, K., Krueger, J., Sureda, B.M., ... Leyden, J. (2005). HER1/EGFR inhibitor-associated rash: Future directions for management and investigation outcomes from the HER1/EGFR inhibitor rash management forum. *Oncologist, 10,* 345–356. doi:10.1634/theoncologist.10-5-345

Porzio, G., Aielli, F., Verna, L., Porto, C., Tudini, M., Cannita, K., & Ficorella, C. (2006). Efficacy of pregabalin in the management of cetuximab-related itch. *Journal of Pain and Symptom Management, 32,* 397–398. doi:10.1016/j.jpainsymman.2006.07.006

Pyle, L., Beirne, D., Bird, J., Hoggarth, L., Jamieson, C., Lane, L., ... Woods, J. (2008). Managing the side effects of sunitinib: A guide to empowering the patient. *Cancer Nursing Practice, 7,* 42–47.

Racca, P., Fanchini, L., Caliendo, V., Ritorto, G., Evangelista, W., Volpatto, R., ... Ciuffreda, L. (2008). Efficacy and skin toxicity management with cetuximab in metastatic colorectal cancer: Outcomes from an oncologic/dermatologic cooperation. *Clinical Colorectal Cancer, 7,* 48–54.

Robert, C., Soria, J.C., & Chosidow, O. (2006). Folliculitis and perionyxis associated with the EGFR inhibitor erlotinib. *Targeted Oncology, 1,* 100–103. doi:10.1007/s11523-006-0013-6

Rose, P.G., Maxson, J.H., Fusco, N., Mossbruger, K., & Rodriguez, M. (2001). Liposomal doxorubicin in ovarian, peritoneal, and tubal carcinoma: A retrospective comparative study of single-agent dosages. *Gynecologic Oncology, 82,* 323–328. doi:10.1006/gyno.2001.6272

Saif, M.W., Elfiky, A., & Diasio, R. (2007). Hand-foot syndrome variant in a dihydropyrimidine dehydrogenase-deficient patient treated with capecitabine. *Clinical Colorectal Cancer, 6,* 219–223.

Scheithauer, W., & Blum, J. (2004). Coming to grips with hand-foot syndrome: Insights from clinical trials evaluating capecitabine. *Oncology, 18,* 1161–1168, 1173.

Scope, A., Agero, A.L., Dusza, S.W., Myskowski, P.L., Lieb, J.A., Saltz, L., ... Halpern, A.C. (2007). Randomized double-blind trial of prophylactic oral minocycline and topical tazarotene for cetuximab-associated acne-like eruption. *Journal of Clinical Oncology, 25,* 5390–5396. doi:10.1200/JCO.2007.12.6987

Segaert, S., Tabernero, J., Chosidow, O., Dirschka, T., Elsner, J., Mancini, L., ... Layton, A. (2005). The management of skin reactions in cancer patients receiving epidermal growth factor receptor targeted therapies. *Journal of the German Society of Dermatology, 3,* 599–606. doi:10.1111/j.1610-0387.2005.05058.x

Segaert, S., & Van Cutsem, E. (2005). Clinical signs, pathophysiology and management of skin toxicity during therapy with epidermal growth factor receptor inhibitors. *Annals of Oncology, 16,* 1425–1433. doi:10.1093/annonc/mdi279

Shah, N.T., Kris, M.G., Pao, W., Tyson, L.B., Pizzo, B.M., Heinemann, M.H., ... Miller, V.A. (2005). Practical management of patients with non-small-cell lung cancer treated with gefitinib. *Journal of Clinical Oncology, 23,* 165–174. doi:10.1200/JCO.2005.04.057

Sipples, R. (2006). Common side effects of anti-EGFR therapy: Acneform rash. *Seminars in Oncology Nursing, 22,* 28–34. doi:10.1016/j.soncn.2006.01.013

Suh, K.Y., Kindler, H.L., Medenica, M., & Lacouture, M. (2006). Doxycycline for the treatment of paronychia induced by the epidermal growth factor receptor inhibitor cetuximab. *British Journal of Dermatology, 154,* 191–192. doi:10.1111/j.1365-2133.2005.07010.x

Swenson, K.K., & Bell, E.M. (2010). Hand-foot syndrome related to liposomal doxorubicin. *Oncology Nursing Forum, 37,* 137–139. doi:10.1188/10.ONF.137-139

Tan, E.H., & Chan, A. (2009). Evidence-based treatment options for the management of skin toxicities associated with epidermal growth factor receptor inhibitors. *Annals of Pharmacology, 43,* 1658–1666. doi:10.1345/aph.1M241

Tanyi, J.L., Smith, J.A., Ramos, L., Parker, C.L., Munsell, M.F., & Wolf, J.K. (2009). Predisposing risk factors for palmar-plantar erythrodesia when using liposomal doxyrubicin to treat recurrent ovarian cancer. *Gynecologic Oncology, 114,* 219–224. doi:10.1016/j.ygyno.2009.04.007

Tedjarati, S., Sayer, R., Boulware, D., & Apte, S. (2006, October). Regional cooling protocol (RCP) significantly reduces the incidence of pegylated liposomal doxorubicin (PLD) induced palmar-plantar erythrodysesthesias (PPE) in patients with recurrent epithelial ovarian cancer [Abstract 302]. Poster presented at the 11th Biennial International Gynecologic Cancer Society Meeting, Santa Monica, CA.

CHAPTER 5. SKIN REACTIONS 121

Titgan, M.A. (1997). Palmar-plantar erythrodysesthesia associated with liposomal encapsulated doxorubicin (Doxil) by oral dexamethasone. *Journal of Clinical Oncology, 16*(Suppl.), Abstract 288. Retrieved from http://www.asco.org/ASCOv2/Meetings/Abstracts?&vmview=abst_detail_view&confID=30&abstractID=11113

Van Doorn, R., Kirtschig, G., Scheffer, E., Stoof, T.J., & Giaccone, G. (2002). Follicular and epidermal alterations in patients treated with ZD1839 (Iressa), an inhibitor of the epidermal growth factor receptor. *British Journal of Dermatology, 147,* 598–601. doi:10.1046/j.1365-2133.2002.04864.x

Vezzoli, P., Marzano, A.V., Onida, F., Alessi, E., Galassi, B., Tomirotti, M., & Berti, E. (2008). Cetuximab-induced acneiform eruption and the response to isotretinoin. *Acta Dermato-Venereologica, 88,* 84–88. doi:10.2340/00015555-0330

Viale, P.H. (2006). Chemotherapy and cutaneous toxicities: Implications for oncology nurses. *Seminars in Oncology Nursing, 22,* 144–151. doi:10.1016/j.soncn.2006.04.007

Vukelja, S.J., Baker, W.J., Burris, H.A., III, Keeling, J.H., & Von Hoff, D. (1993). Pyridoxine therapy for palmar-plantar erythrodysesthesia associated with Taxotere. *Journal of the National Cancer Institute, 85,* 1432–1433.

Wagner, L.I., & Lacouture, M.E. (2007). Dermatologic toxicities associated with EGFR inhibitors: The clinical psychologist's perspective. Impact on health-related quality of life and implications for clinical management of psychological sequelae. *Oncology, 21*(11, Suppl. 5), 34–36.

Webster-Gandy, J.D., How, C., & Harrold, K. (2007). Palmar-plantar erythrodysesthesia (PPE): A literature review with commentary on experience in a cancer centre. *European Journal of Oncology Nursing, 11,* 238–246. doi:10.1016/j.ejon.2006.10.004

Wilkes, G.M., & Doyle, D. (2005). Palmar-plantar erythrodysesthesia. *Clinical Journal of Oncology Nursing, 9,* 103–106. doi:10.1188/05.CJON.103-106

Zimmerman, G.C., Keeling, J.H., Lowry, M., Medina, J., Von Hoff, D.D., & Burris, H.A. (1994). Prevention of docetaxel-induced erythrodysesthesia with local hypothermia. *Journal of the National Cancer Institute, 86,* 557–558. doi:10.1093/jnci/86.7.557

Index

The letter f after a page number indicates that relevant content appears in a figure; the letter t, in a table.

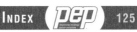

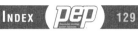